CRUCIBLE OF THE INCURABLE

EXPERTISE

**CULTURES AND
TECHNOLOGIES
OF KNOWLEDGE**

EDITED BY DOMINIC BOYER

A list of titles in this series is available at cornellpress.cornell.edu.

CRUCIBLE OF THE INCURABLE

Facing ALS

Anthony Stavrianakis

CORNELL UNIVERSITY PRESS   ITHACA AND LONDON

First published 2024 by Cornell University Press

Library of Congress Cataloging-in-Publication Data

Names: Stavrianakis, Anthony, author.
Title: Crucible of the incurable : facing ALS / Anthony Stavrianakis.
Description: Ithaca : Cornell University Press, 2024. | Series: Expertise: cultures and technologies of knowledge | Includes bibliographical references and index.
Identifiers: LCCN 2024022411 (print) | LCCN 2024022412 (ebook) | ISBN 9781501778315 (hardcover) | ISBN 9781501778322 (paperback) | ISBN 9781501778339 (epub) | ISBN 9781501778346 (pdf)
Subjects: LCSH: Amyotrophic lateral sclerosis—Patients—Social conditions. | Amyotrophic lateral sclerosis—Psychological aspects. | Amyotrophic lateral sclerosis—Patients—Care.
Classification: LCC RC406.A24 S78 2024 (print) | LCC RC406.A24 (ebook) | DDC 616.8/39—dc23/eng/20240613
LC record available at https://lccn.loc.gov/2024022411
LC ebook record available at https://lccn.loc.gov/2024022412

For Gwen

Contents

FACING AMYOTROPHIC LATERAL SCLEROSIS

The work for this book began as a set of addenda. From 2013 through 2017, I had been conducting an inquiry in Switzerland on the practice of assisted suicide. I was trying to accompany people as they reflected on whether to ask for help with voluntarily ending their lives. During that research, the results of which were subsequently published in 2020 as *Leaving: A Narrative of Assisted Suicide*, I met many people who were living with amyotrophic lateral sclerosis (ALS), enduring it to different degrees. ALS is a progressive neurodegenerative disease that affects nerve cells in the brain and spinal cord. I had also met friends and family of people who were affected by ALS, who narrated to me their experience of the illness, and particularly the decisions of their loved ones to end their lives. I knew from available statistics for Switzerland that, proportionally speaking, neurodegenerative diseases comprise the most frequent diagnostic category for requests for assistance with suicide. Since my objective was to understand how people work through their experiences of life and illness and come to a judgment to end their lives with assistance from others, ALS was just one illness among others that constituted an underlying reason for their asking for help.

At that time, I was not really concerned with the different ways that people reflected on living and dying when confronted with this specific illness. I was not concerned with the multiplicity of practices of preparing for the end of life when voluntary death was only one way among others. I did not know very much about the illness, beyond the fragments of life that were shared with me as reason, as cause, so to speak, for wishing to leave it. The well filled slowly. An aggregate of notes and fragments, which I did not know what to do with, were filed away.

A preoccupation persisted, however: How do people live with ALS, and how do they live with others while living with it? How is the person suffering with the illness attended to by others, and how do they attend to themselves? Such a form of attention is sometimes called "care." What does that term signify when it concerns a diagnosis of a chronic, currently 100 percent fatal, neuromuscular neurodegenerative illness? How do people diagnosed with ALS continue to live as well as possible, for as long as possible? These questions stemmed from a solicitude about the lives of those I had met, which had given me a nascent impression of how singularly, or specifically, cruel the illness can be, as well as the heterogeneity of ways of facing, working over, and working through the experience of this illness.

Perhaps these were simply, not to say merely, some chance encounters with people whose stories were troubling, stories that were preoccupying and affecting. Yet I thought they were more than that. I could not shake the thought that my preoccupation with the illness had something to do not only with the people I had met but with the illness itself. Or rather, to put it more accurately, what this particular illness makes visible for and about people.

Instances: Peter, a British man whom I wrote about in *Leaving*, had held a lifelong obsession, and fear, of developing a locked-in syndrome. At age seventy-one, he was diagnosed with "motor neuron disease," the British term for the range of progressive neurodegenerative illnesses that are called ALS in the United States. Gaby, the devout Catholic in the canton of Valais in Switzerland, who surprised everyone after hearing the diagnosis, on learning the likely trajectory of the illness, the impossibility of repair, by turning to her husband to say that she would not stay for the end, and made him promise her, in front of the doctor, to help her leave in peace, which he did, and which she did. Jean-Marc, the rough, tough phone repairman, in the Cantal in France, whose diagnosis of ALS had spurred reflection on his abusive past and provided the turning point to ask for forgiveness from his children, with whom he had had no contact in decades. Repair by way of the impossibility of repair.

Any illness could be said to be a test. The thought that endured, however, was that there is something specific about ALS. I cannot prove this, whatever that might mean, and I certainly will not try to. Despite what I have heard and read repeatedly about ALS, there is no "worst disease." ALS is one among other terrible illnesses. What I could do, and did do, however, was to spend several years learning about the illness and to spend a year doing fieldwork, meeting people who in different ways are concerned with the illness, to try to discern what about it had been preoccupying me.

It was roughly in 2016 that I began to think about all this. Laurence Tessier, who was studying the diagnosis and medical management of cerebral and neurological illnesses, suggested we write a grant proposal together. In our discussions and through writing the proposal, we aimed to bring our two areas of concern into a common framing: the diagnosis and the ways of managing the symptoms of patients diagnosed with different kinds of neurological and cerebral affliction.[1] I proposed to work on ALS and she would work with people, and with the families of those, diagnosed with Alzheimer's disease, as well as those admitted to neurointensive care. We decided that Northern California would be a good place for the inquiry. We were familiar with the area and with a number of the academic and medical institutions there, and we had a strong desire to return, having both been graduate students in the region.

We left Paris for the academic year August 2019–June 2020, funded for eleven months of fieldwork by the Agence National de la Recherche. We were hosted as visiting researchers at a local teaching university. Through this position, I was able to make contact with two distinct and interconnected field sites: an ALS clinic and an outpatient noncancer palliative care clinic, located in the same medical center. It is noteworthy that just as I arrived in California, the latter clinic had been made a permanent institutional fixture, in addition to the inpatient palliative care team and outpatient cancer palliative care team, after a trial period of several years. It is also worth considering that this noncancer outpatient palliative care clinic had started as part of the ALS clinic, and it is important to note that their patient population is roughly one-quarter ALS. The institutional arrangement is not unique, but it is exemplary of the overlap between ALS clinical management and palliative care consultations. Moreover, the organizational arrangement exemplified the perceived need for increased access to palliative care for illnesses other than cancer.

Access to these sites afforded me the opportunity to observe the diagnosis of ALS, to follow quarterly visits in which the progression of the illness is monitored and to see how physical, social, and environmental needs of the person are considered, as well as how conversations with palliative care teams about psychophysical symptoms and goals of care are conducted. Through clinical observation, I could grasp what current multidisciplinary care involves at one nationally recognized center.

More broadly, my aim was to track what happens after diagnosis is made, understand what "symptom management" options are available for patients, and listen to how patients and their families make use of these available options within a broader effort to live with this progressive neurodegenerative disease. By spending time with people who have been diagnosed with ALS, I wished to describe how different kinds of work or interventions on the body, on the home and on the social environment of the patient, as well as with the person, are connected to goals, purposes, and aims of care, as understood by the patient and those who live with them and look after them, if and when such rationalized (means–ends) action is taken. Furthermore, it is crucial to attend to those moments when patients or families are unable or unwilling to engage in proposed management and refuse the techniques and interventions offered.

Important to underscore, and this will be a key historical element of this work, is that "rationalized" ALS care, by which I mean the presentation of a range of possible interventions for the patient with ALS correlated to the advancement of the illness and the particular circumstances of the person, is historically (relatively) new: the key date I will provide is 1975. Hence, it is important to realize that such management was not always an obvious manner of responding medically to the illness, for patients and for medical staff. As I will explain at length, since the identification of the specificity of this illness in 1870, there has been only a tiny change in what medicine can offer in terms of slowing down the progression of this illness—a drug that seems to provide, on average, two to three extra months of life. Within this situation, whose ultimate reality has not changed, rationalized multidisciplinary management was an intervention, developed at the intersection of neurology, nursing, new considerations of palliative care, nutrition counseling, social work, and spiritual care, from roughly 1975, starting in the United States.

Such a model of illness management, which transformed a diagnosis of a fatal degenerative illness into a chronic and evolving degenerative set of specific disabilities (difficulties with movement, eating, and speech, among others) slowly became the normative orientation for medical practice concerning ALS. This was in contrast to what was, up until then, a hands-off approach, one that had been in place globally up until the early 1970s. The medical ethical orientation that was normative prior to the 1970s claimed that the most humane thing to do for people with ALS was to do nothing, so as not to prolong suffering with this illness. Such an approach meant also, for the medical professional, not to have to face, face up to, the limits of medical cure and the question of what care is possible and appropriate when there is no treatment to reverse or halt the progression of the illness.

ALS in California

Although it was not a principal focus of the inquiry, one reason for wanting to do the project in California was that a bill in support of "medical aid in dying" had been passed, which became a state law in 2016: the California End of Life Option Act (EOLOA). As such, I could observe how "medical aid in dying," the Californian term for assisted suicide, was considered as one option among others for people living with ALS. It became a possible way to end an experience of suffering, as illness progressed. The motivation was not for this inquiry to be a "part b" to a project already concluded, in which I would compare Californian aid in dying with Swiss assisted suicide, although there are intriguing and notable differences. I wanted rather to focus on the illness itself, knowledge of the illness as lived by those who have some form of experience with it, in a situation in which at least two things are present: support for those diagnosed with ALS through multidisciplinary clinics and a legally available "option" to end one's life once the illness has progressed to a six-month prognosis. If a certain number of people made the decision to leave their experience of ALS, something that was certainly possible even before the passing of the state legislation to allow physician-assisted suicide and takes on a distinct form in the guise of medical aid in dying, others, the vast majority of people, it must be stated, continue to live until the forces pushing against death are overwhelmed by the illness.

ALS, as I will endeavor to show, has a specific "sense of certitude" about it, to take up Jean-Martin Charcot's (1825–1893) phrase, despite its variations and despite (and also because of) the indetermination as to the biology of its cause. The sense(s) and affect(s) of certitude are in play for all who are confronted with it. The illness is 100 percent fatal. It is common for the duration of the illness to last between two and five years. Twenty percent of people live five years or more, and 10 percent ten years or more, postdiagnosis. During that time, the body loses certain capacities, bit by bit. The person living with the illness endeavors to live with these losses, to impose their own vitality and normativity amid the discordance. It is for these two reasons, the senses of certitude and the indetermination as to its cause, as well as its clinical presentation, that I think there is something specific, although not unique, about this illness. Creutzfeldt–Jakob disease (CJD) would be another case of an illness—in this case, a prion disease, a misfolded protein that can transmit its misfolded shape to other normal versions of the same protein—that is universally fatal, has both familial (genetic) and sporadic variants, and is able to be transmitted through other means, for instance, tainted growth hormones.[2] One difference worth bearing in mind is that the cause of CJD, like Huntington's, is known. When faced with these aspects of ALS concerning certitude and indetermination, no doubt shared with other universally fatal illnesses, a question presents itself as to how a person bears this knowledge and the experience of the illness, a question of countenance, and of how to countenance and work through and grasp the challenges, the losses, and the moments of enjoyment in life after the diagnosis.

Countenance. As a noun, it points to the question of how each person, how any person, how you or I would be, and how we would live, when faced with a situation of this kind. And countenance as a verb: what will you countenance, how will you support, what will be tolerated, and to what end?

I came across the term "countenance" in a set of letters that I will recount later in the book—letters dating from the period 1974–1979, a historical moment that is key to the narrative of this book, written by a person living with ALS, Frances McGill. Born in the twentieth century but raised in the (style of the) nineteenth, a friend of hers wrote at the start of a published book of letters about her experience. This child of a medical missionary family raised in Turkey, Ms. McGill wrote the following about the experience of paralysis due to her illness, dictated by way of Morse code expressed solely through the exhausting and time-consuming movements of her eyes:

> When one's identity is diminished to near zero, and one's energy is near minus and one is confined to a bed in the same room day after day, one's perspective changes, and everything seems to revolve around one's pain and anxiety and lost hopes. So it was that I could believe that all over-heard conversations were about me, and all countenances expressed feelings emanating from attitudes toward me. So the whole world re-volves around me. I was almost as innocent as a new born baby in this respect.[3]

There is a lot in these sentences, and I will endeavor to unpack it later in the book. For now, let me simply say that her choice of the word "countenances" gave me pause for thought as I read the passage and sent me to the dictionary.

The countenances in question in her letter are both of those who were around her and of her own awareness of her own attitude, her poise and bearing: this, I thought to myself, was absolutely right. There is something specific about try-ing to face people who are themselves facing this specific illness. It's not about facing up to "death," as though that was not impossible. The problem is more nuanced than that: it's about how to face, to countenance, the face and counte-nance of the one with this illness, an illness with an expected set of cruelties as well as its heterogeneous, and surprising, expressions. Insofar as it is a progres-sive degenerative disease that currently can be slowed by approximately three months, the outcome is thought to be, to a large degree, known in advance. With time, physical functions will cease. Which one is next? How long will it take? These are the dependent variables. There is time to prepare, but it is only in the encounters with medical knowledge and technique, the contours of everyday life at home, and the concern and expectations about what one will become and how one will become that a person's countenance is rendered visible and not as some-thing already given.

There are longstanding traditions in the social sciences, the humanities, and philosophy of what, following Kenneth Burke, could broadly be called "litera-ture as equipment for living" or what he calls the "sociological criticism of liter-ature,"[4] of which sociology or anthropology itself can be a medium through which to learn something about how to face life lived within the knots of social relations, with a body subject to constraint and loss, with margins of freedom to invent ways of doing, and speaking and writing, when confronted with such loss.[5] I can but gesture to the fact that I consider anthropology to be just such an "equipment," a means of tracking, in this case, how people confront and give form to one of the reals of an existence, finitude.

Two Images

The term "countenance" resonated with two vivid images, which have stayed with me over the years—images conjured through the words of those who loved them, regarding people who had suffered with ALS, both of them French, who lived in Paris.

October 2017: I walked to Nathalie's place. By chance, we lived close to each other, where rue de Rochechouart in the ninth arrondissement almost touches the boulevard Barbès in the eighteenth. The calm of her apartment was accentuated by the rising sound of children playing in a schoolyard, their cries and cackles swirling up on the warm waves of autumn air, echoing among the shadows of the trees and leaves of the cool court below, floating in through the window, out of which the smoke of her cigarette whirled.

This was not the first time I have wondered about why I was doing this, collecting sad stories, and grief, leaving with words in a notebook, impressions, images. As Emma, one of the people whom you will read about in this book, put it to me, the first time we met, the only way having this illness could make sense to her was by thinking that she was supposed to learn something from it. I endeavored to do the same, without presupposing what I would learn is the same, or that it could or should be limited to the redescription of her (self)-understanding, the self-understanding of others, although such redescription is necessary, obligatory even.

Nathalie and I had been put in touch by an association in Switzerland. She had begun trying to change the law on assistance with suicide and euthanasia in France, eight months after the death of Michel, her husband, who had ALS. Nathalie had started a petition on change.org, addressed to the minister of health, requesting the legalization of active aid in dying (*L'aide active à mourir*), which quickly, within a year, had well over 100,000 signatures and five years later had close to half a million. "I am neither a lawyer nor a militant," she said, as we sat facing each other, "I wished merely to testify eight months after his death from ALS so that the right to assisted suicide exists in France as soon as possible." Despite moments of expectation, as of the time of writing, nothing has changed in France.

Michel's illness started as an iteration of a familiar, sobering set of events: it began with a little trouble lifting his toes, three years before he died. He went to see a rheumatologist and a neurologist in Neuilly, a well-off suburb. A herniated disc, he was told. An operation and physical therapy followed. Nothing changed. Half a year later, he began to fall in the holiday heat of a Greek island and had a serious accident. "ALS cannot be ruled out," the same doctor then told him, in a subsequent email. Michel went to the Pitié-Salpêtrière hospital to find out.

Unable to do all the tests—"I forget which one," Nathalie said, "perhaps the EMG," I said, "yes, perhaps," she replied—he had to wait to feel better before he could finish them all and to know what was happening to him. It took the best part of the autumn and early winter to have a diagnosis, finally announced a few days before Christmas 2011. By spring, a wheelchair. All this time he carried on seeing patients. Michel was a doctor, a psychiatrist and psychoanalyst, specializing in the analysis of children. He had been analyzed by Jacques Lacan (1901–1981) and he had trained with Françoise Dolto (1908–1988).

By the spring, the next episode in a series that cannot be halted, a series told in clear-eyed entirety by Charcot 170 years ago, and told to me by Nathalie: "And then it was his arms. Little by little, we had to renounce all that we loved to do together." Nathalie spoke quickly, perhaps to make it hurt less: walking in Paris, going to the cinema and opera, dancing, cooking together. Opera is not incidental for them. Michel and Nathalie had known each other while Michel was still married to his second wife. They had met through mutual friends, at a dinner. Love forbidden at first sight. They both loved opera, unlike their spouses. The death of Michel's wife, whom he cared for to the end, after a long illness, was what allowed their love to flourish:

> Our love was unconditional, it sustained us during this terrifying test, his body sinking in sand that no hands, neither mine, always in his, nor a doctor's, could do anything to stop. Even as it got worse, though, there were moments of hope, or rather, despite knowing that hope was fanciful, we gathered all our strength at every minute, each of us a support to the other when forlorn. We wanted to believe in a possible hope. And then, it became obvious that death would catch up with us, we two atheists, raised as Christians, who lived our life far from a faith in which some find refuge, perhaps consolation.

Nathalie tells this story, she says, in order to help others understand how at a given moment, a decision to die, what she, like so many others call "a choice," can become the only possible alternative for someone who is ill.

She tells the story, she says, to make that alternative legal, and not only possible, in the country of her birth and Michel's death. I think she also tells the story as a way of trying to repair, perhaps work through, how he actually died with this disease.

In her petition-length version of the narrative, the story is relatively simple: a terrible incurable illness, an unconditional love that couldn't heal, a wish to die at a moment of his choosing, which went unfulfilled because of the reticence of a medical corps that has long sustained through its paternalism a suspicion of individual autonomy.

In Nathalie's rendering, the narrative form is almost tragic, in a strict classical sense: a hero succumbs to an awful fate precisely because of a virtue he tries to uphold. In Michel's case, the strength of his love for Nathalie and his three children, his commitment to his child analysands, the intransigence of the French medical corps, and the strength of her love for him conspired to lock him into a situation in which he would be forced to wait out his death at home and to have Nathalie and his children accompany him through it. His strength, his virtue, became a torment and was his downfall. Her anger is directed at the gods of the medical corp. Unlike the tragic figure, and this is where it departs from the genre strictly speaking, whatever Michel's flaws or vices, they were not the cause of his suffering. There was no choice between having the illness or not. He made a choice, however, to wait until he could bear it no longer, a moment at which it was too late to leave for Switzerland. The illness is what the person encounters, and it is the person who must show their countenance with respect to it.

The story she tells assembles, composes, and compresses, still more layers of their experience. By June 2013, the sign of a turning point had appeared— diaphragmatic involvement. The team at the Salpêtrière asked Michel to consider participation in a phase III phrenic stimulation trial at the hospital, which had begun in 2012. "We both read the information they gave us," Nathalie narrated. "I found it barbaric. We had to go to the sleep center as a first step, an overnight study, and there they didn't even have a chair for him to be able to go to the toilet or to take a shower without someone carrying him. He thought it would give him six more months. Instead, he had postoperative pneumonia. They called me from the ICU but wouldn't let me see him." This was the event that got him to think about assisted suicide. It was mid-October.

The word "thinking" should be highlighted: in Natalie's terms, dying in hospital was something that horrified him. She put it down to his medical training, his experience in neonatal intensive care, and the deaths of his mother, his father, and his second wife. Michel's' mother died a difficult death with Alzheimer's in a hospital ward, and his father was traumatized by World War II and died as an alcoholic in the hospital of cirrhosis of the liver. "He told me 'if it's too difficult [to have me at home] I will go to hospital,' but I had promised him." She points to a pair of sculpted metal Balinese bells:

We had a system, if he needed something, he'd ring. He stayed for me. At his request I contacted three associations in Switzerland, and only one wrote back with a humane reply. Erika, the head, said she was going to be in Paris that weekend, and she came to the house. I had also contacted a person in China who claimed to produce and sell pentobarbital, the lethal medication. The palliative care team at the hospital offered Haldol [an antipsychotic medication]. Michel told them that the only thing he had left were his thoughts, so he didn't want them to take that away from him. He saw his final patient at the end of November. He would use the cough assist machine and an expectorant [to help him breathe] sometimes between two patients. One of the children said to him that they'd like to be a doctor when they grow up, that way they could heal him if he ever got sick.

Erika, the head of the Swiss association, saw that he was in no way able to make the journey to Basel. She was sorry, but it was too late. It was mid-December. Two weeks later, he would be dead:

His breathing was becoming very difficult. He was aware the end was near and he wanted it to end. He wanted a dose of morphine. Just before Christmas, the family doctor would not prescribe it for him. The day after Christmas, the children and I packed up the wheelchair and slowly made our way out of the apartment, down the lift, or rather up and down the lift so many times to take first the chair, then the bags, then Michel, and on to the hospital. Neurology couldn't see him, the ALS center couldn't see him, finally he was seen in the ER. A prescription for morphine was given to him, but I could only collect it the next day from the pharmacy. We waited three hours for an ambulance home. That night he began having serious problems breathing. He had already had such a bout of respiratory failure. At the time I had asked him, if he has this kind of trouble breathing again, does he want me to do the same thing [i.e., save his life]. He had said no. He was on the floor of the kitchen, and I let him go. The last thing I said to him was *je te laisse* [I'm letting you go].

Nathalie introduced me to Georges, whose wife Jacqueline had died with ALS. He lived in her neighborhood. Two people with ALS in the ninth arrondissement of Paris. One of the most common of the rare diseases. Statistically four to six cases per 100,000. The ninth has a population of 60,000. So they were the two for the arrondissement for 2011–2013. Since they died, two others will have had to take their place, and then two more. What connects Georges and Na-thalie is not only the illness but that Georges's wife, Jacqueline, was able to die the way that Nathalie says that Michel wished to die. I put it this way as a matter of fidelity to the situation. I only spoke with Nathalie, not Michel; moreover, I put it this way because of what I learned previously by inquiring into assisted suicide as a practice: while many people say they are in favor of it, in favor of personal freedom and choice et cetera, and while a small number of people who are actually ill do ask for assistance with suicide, only half of that small num-ber go through with it.

Most people, as has been well documented, are reassured simply by the idea that they have the option of ending their suffering if they wish to. Most people do not do it. Michel did not look for, apparently didn't wish to have, that reas-surance while he was living with ALS. It was once he was in the actual process of dying that he, and his family, began to look for a way out and created the con-ditions in which they could both look for that way out together and find a target for the anger for the way in which he died: a recalcitrant, ill-equipped medical corps. Michel could remain who he had been: a loving father and husband who stayed to the end, who suffered for the sake of love and commitment.

Jacqueline's death was very different, although it began in much the same way. A holiday in Normandy, a fall on a walk by the sea. Very strange. Everyone else ignored it, said it was nothing. But she took note, as was her wont. She was ex-tremely sharp. A person of great intelligence, the doctor's report for the assisted suicide organization in Switzerland stated. She has an absolute conviction in her values, the same letter concluded. One of those values was knowledge and the form it takes in learning, as well as an unbridled curiosity. Another was secrecy, something she shared with her neighbor and close friend, a philosopher who lived a few floors above Jacqueline, Georges, and their daughter Veronique. Knowledge. She figured it out pretty quickly. She had taken note, and notes, co-pious notes, of what was happening to her. The fall, then a little difficulty with the toes. Some stiffness. "Oh you've been talking to Dr. Google," a neurologist condescended to her. A year later, the progression of the symptoms and the EMG result made it difficult for the medical corps not to concur with her. This was not her first serious illness. Jacqueline had worked through a lot of illness in her life before being diagnosed with ALS: a hysterectomy (their daughter came to them through adoption), a double pulmonary embolism, and an aggressive breast cancer. Secrecy. When she was diagnosed with cancer, it was the philosopher's sister who had taken care of her, a very good surgeon. The philosopher had died already six years previously, having ended his life. He had encouraged Jacque-line to write. She wrote only for herself, though. It was her teaching that was public. Her skill as a Spanish teacher was matched by her curiosity and love of youth. Georges sketched an image for me: he had come back to the apartment one day, after running a quick errand. Jacqueline had an enormous smile on her face. She hadn't looked that joyous in a while. Midst an apartment full of books, paintings, and sculptures, Jaqueline was gesturing toward the screen in front of her. She wrote on the board that she used to communicate with, since her tongue could no longer form speech: "look, it's great!" She had found the latest video from the pop singer Maître Gims, and the video she was playing was "*J'me tire*" ("I'm outta here").

Given what had happened to their philosopher neighbor, given his suicide, Jacqueline thought that his sister would help her. Jacqueline wasn't going to stay to the end. She had already thought about suicide in 2005, in case she was unable to be cured of the cancer. In 2012, she became a member of the French Association for the Right to Die with Dignity (ADMD). Jacqueline took an appointment with her, and she promised Jacqueline that when the time comes, "we'll help you." The illness progressed. She refused to take her meals with her husband and daughter. Self-exclusion. She wouldn't accept having a feeding tube and so ate slowly by making her food into a paste. Georges says, matter of factly, that he understood why she kept herself apart at mealtimes. They couldn't pretend that things hadn't changed, and eating separately was a way, their way, of facing the situation, of marking loss. A little stool to help her shower had to be changed to a larger device to fulfill the same function. And then: she'd had enough. They went back to see the philosopher's sister. She said she'd take care of it. They received a phone call from Jeanne Garnier, a hospice. Entering the hospice, she passed a chapel within the institution, a figure of Jesus lit so as to cast a large striking shadow.

"I want you to help me," she wrote on her little board. "We can't do that," the hospice staff said. She asked them to call the philosopher's sister, who spoke with the staff, who then reported back. "What are you going to do?" Georges asked them. "We'll take care of her," said the staff. "But we can't do anything [i.e., hasten death] *until she is like this*," the hospice physician said, making a gesture of the head falling to one side, an uncontrolled grimace locked on the face.

"Get me out of here" appeared on Jacqueline's writing board.

Georges told me that they then took her home and phoned the family doctor. "You left the Rolls Royce of hospice care!" the family doctor exclaimed.

He did, however, agree to prescribe morphine. Georges was incredulous: "What was I supposed to do with this? I've never injected anything in my life. Was I supposed to take responsibility for this?"

Erika from the Swiss association was back in Paris the weekend that Jacqueline left the hospice. Veronique went to her talk at the Paris offices of the Right to Die Association and somehow, she said, mustered the courage to approach her. Erika agreed to visit Jacqueline at home and saw that she was determined, had thought about it, and, crucially, could make the journey. A long, exhausting ambulance ride from Paris to Basel. Veronique offered her a copy of *Libé*, but she waved it away. She asked her what she was doing: "reciting poetry to myself," Jacqueline replied.

Acknowledgments

With the publication of this book, I am bringing to a close a period of inquiry that began in 2019 with the encouragement, goodwill, and kind collaboration of the two Californian clinics that I have called, so as to preserve anonymity, "ALS clinic" and "palliative care clinic." I am deeply grateful to the clinicians working in these two sites who provided an environment in which to observe their practice, to ask questions, and to draw out the nuances of clinical care for ALS. I am moreover very grateful to those patients who took the time to talk with me, to the person I have called Emma and especially to Gwen Petersen and Nathan Petersen, for whom I gladly wave the principle of anonymity in respect of an ethic of recognition. I would like to thank the Agence nationale de recherche (ANR ANR-17-CE36–0007) in France for their financial support, the administrative staff at the institutions in California for their assistance, and the staff at my home institution, the CNRS, particularly Farida Djeridi.

The writing of this book was kept in motion through conversations with a number of friends. I would like to thank Talia Dan-Cohen, Bharat Venkat, Todd Meyers, and Robert Desjarlais. In Paris, I owe a big debt to Nicolas Dodier, whose mentorship since I arrived in 2013 has been invaluable. The "petit groupe" at the EHESS was an important part of testing out a late version of several parts of the book, and thus I would like to thank Janine Barbot, Michel Naepels, Stefan Le Courant, and Catherine Rémy for our numerous conversations, as well as Vololona Rabeharisoa, Myriam Winance, and Gregory Delaplace for their thoughtful engagement with the manuscript. I had the occasion to present an outline of the project to the Department of Anthropology research seminar at Oxford University; my sincere thanks to Anthony Howarth, Elizabeth Hallam, and Thomas Cousins for our discussion. At Cornell University Press, I am very fortunate to have encountered Dominic Boyer and Jim Lance, whose interest and support for the book project was a boon.

The ethnography for the book was conducted from August 2019 to June 2020, which included a period rife with indetermination and discordance. I would like to thank Laurence Tessier and Marcel Stavrianakis; it was a pretty good year, *malgré tout*.

Lastly, a word in memory of Paul Rabinow, with whom week in and week out over the course of that year, like the ten years before that, I would test what I was doing. That work has come to end, and so it's time to start again.

ON LINKING KNOWLEDGE AND CARE FOR ALS

The object and objective of this book is to grasp how people invent forms, techniques, and practices for living with a universally fatal neurodegenerative illness, amyotrophic lateral sclerosis (ALS). Living with this illness implies knowledge about it, which is to say that which people are confronted with when they encounter a diagnosis and the medical discourse that accompanies their experience of it. There is also a normative concern, on the part of medical practitioners, friends, families, and patients themselves, about how one should care for, and be cared for, when living with this illness. And there is the question of the specificity of the way that each person diagnosed gives form to a life once this illness becomes a part of it.

More specifically, concerning forms of knowledge about ALS, what matters are the determinations and indeterminations in how signs of illness are arranged. There is a curious doubling in knowledge and ignorance about ALS: clinically, since 1875, there has been a certitude of diagnosis, accompanied nevertheless by serious indeterminations concerning etiology and nosology. With respect to the normative concern about conduct, I will focus on explicit and implicit evaluations at play in clinical apparatuses, in multidisciplinary ALS clinics and palliative care clinics that support and care for people with the illness, making use of available knowledge. Specifically, I will show how work in these clinics at different moments takes up evaluative questions linked to technical concerns of medical management, management of body functions, preoccupations about identity linked to those functions, issues of personhood, and questions concerning how to approach the fact of the universal fatality of the illness, the issue of dying. With respect to the question of giving form to a life with ALS, I take this up in terms of how individuals use mediums of language, writing, talking, and "giving voice," as ways, their own, of working through their experience of living with ALS.

ALS as an Object of Inquiry in the Social Sciences

Since 2014, there have been a few and increasing number of studies in the social sciences that have taken up ALS management, as well as the lives of people living with this illness, as an object of inquiry. These studies can be broadly organized into three groups, which partly overlap. First, there are studies, inspired by social studies of science and technology, that look very closely at the technical interventions and tools that come to matter for those who have ALS. Jeannette Pols, a Dutch researcher specializing in the empirical study of ethics, along with medical colleagues in the Netherlands, has been a forerunner in this work, looking at how people with ALS make choices and navigate options in terms of bodily interventions, notably concerning feeding tubes, breathing apparatuses, and end-of-life care.[1] A second area of work has taken a "narrative" approach to experiences with ALS, of which a key researcher has been the Cardiff-based Dikaios Sakellariou, whose work sits at the intersection of medical sociology, public health, disability studies, and occupational therapy.[2] A third approach, forged by the US anthropologist and public health scholar Chelsea Carter, has focused on uncovering discriminatory effects of racial representations in ALS diagnosis and specifically "biases in ALS epistemic paradigms."[3]

I am aware of these approaches without necessarily fitting into any single one of them. Moreover, I found it necessary to combine an anthropological account grounded in observations and discussions in the present with historical work, thus connecting this book to available work in the history of medicine and specifically the history of neurology. It is worth noting that neurology as a medical specialty has a curious characteristic of being one of the medical specialties with a particular historical awareness. Indeed, most historical studies of amyotrophic lateral sclerosis and connected neuromuscular diseases have been conducted by physician-historians. Unlike studies of things such as cognitive disorders and conversion syndromes (hysteria), which have been objects of study for cultural historians, sociologists, anthropologists, and the like, neuromuscular illness has tended to be a specialist concern for historically minded neurologists.

Despite the relatively restricted number of works specifically on ALS, it is possible to look at several neurological illnesses that share some characteristics with ALS to situate this book. Moreover, it is possible to look beyond neurological illnesses: transmissible illnesses with universal or near-universal fatality, such as rabies, transmissible spongiform encephalopathies, or visceral leishmaniasis, or else forms of cancer with very poor prognosis, such as pancreatic or ovarian cancer. The choice of situating an anthropological study in relation to social scientific work on several other neurological illnesses, not all of which have such a poor prognosis, stems from two sources: first, that despite their heterogeneous clinical presentation, neurodegenerative illnesses share features in terms of how care can be provided, especially regarding motor degeneration symptoms, and, second, that neurological illnesses are characterized by the fact that knowledge about them is in a deeply asymmetrical relation to the care that can be provided for those suffering with them. It is this relation between knowledge and care that I think justifies situating a study of ALS in relation to other neurodegenerative illnesses. I will thus briefly outline how other researchers in the social sciences have taken up illnesses such as muscular dystrophies, Huntington's disease, multiple sclerosis, and Parkinson's disease.

Social Scientific Inquiries into Neurodegenerative Illnesses

Over the course of roughly a decade, beginning in the late 1990s, Vololona Rabeharisoa and Michel Callon developed a distinctive research program concerning the involvement of patients diagnosed with myopathies in the research activities (financially) supported by the Association française contre les myopathies.[4] The broad set of research concerns established by Rabeharisoa and Callon includes the emerging relations between social identities, genetic knowledge, and medical–genetic testing; the interlinking of research programs and political debate, specifically in connection to the emerging social identities of patients with respect to genetic and medical research; and the involvement of patient groups in orienting research programs. It was crucial for Rabeharisoa and Callon to observe identity formation, in the nexus of science and politics, as an achievement, rather than as a starting point. The connection to ALS can be made explicit: in the work of muscular dystrophy activists, the social existence of patients and their entourage was mediated both by participation in research, as objects of study, and through an emergent apparatus of recognition—the recognition of patients as "full-fledged persons by the professions that normally cared for and helped patients and as citizens in their own right."[5] A key event, noted by the sociologists, was the International Classification of Impairments, Disabilities and Handicaps, 1976. Crucially, there is motion between these two modes of existence (that of being a patient and a citizen). On the one hand, there is what Callon has called the "framing" of orphan diseases, in which a patient is recognized with certain rights but within which the parameters of research are relatively fixed, which becomes a problem when dealing with diseases whose basic prognosis has not changed over centuries. On the other hand, there is what he calls "overflowing," which occurs when different people take up externalities, concerns, problems, information, connected practices, and so on, which are outside or spill out from the way that a given set of practices is framed.[6] To give an example that I will return to in the very last chapter of this book—an instance of "overflow" from the "framing" of ALS as an orphan disease—a new "patient-centered movement" for ALS called I AM ALS has oriented its work, in part, by a claim drawing on emerging scientific research that there are likely to be connected molecular pathological pathways that link ALS with other illnesses such as frontotemporal dementia, Parkinson's, and Huntington's, such that a "cure for one" (one disease, one body) is a "cure for all" (a set of interconnected diseases and the bodies affected by them). I AM ALS endeavors to enact precisely the kind of patient expertise and emergent social identity that Rabeharisoa and Callon studied in the context of the myopathies, remediating how research agendas are forged and producing new arrangements for those living with ALS, arrangements of patients, families, clinical trial apparatuses, clinical apparatuses, funders, biotech startups, off-label and nonstandard treatments, technologies, and so on. The work of this organization can be contrasted with "ALSA," the long-standing ALS Association, which is considered by some patients, especially those who have invested time and energy into other avenues of work, as being a slow-moving organization that is not calibrated to the urgency of a demand and a desire for patients to participate in research, to try to access new therapies, and to connect the work of an organization to the temporal horizon of their own illness, even if critics do acknowledge that ALSA itself recognizes the need for such participation.

With respect to Huntington's, we have a case in point of individuals diagnosed with this illness not only participating in medicoscientific research programs but also forming their own institutions for the coproduction of knowledge about both illness and the disease, to wit, the Franco-Belgian Institute *Dingdingdong*. It was founded in 2012 and is run by Emilie Hermant and Valérie Pihet, along with a range of artists, social scientists, philosophers, and a neurologist:

> *Dingdingdong*'s challenge is to establish a system of knowledge production that articulates the collection of individual accounts with the development of new pragmatic proposals, with a view to helping its users (*usagers*)—carriers, patients, kin, caregivers—to live with Huntington's

honorably. Original forms of collaboration between users, researchers (medicine, philosophy, sociology, history), and artists (fine artists, writers, videographers, choreographers...) are needed for an endeavor such as this: probing this disease as unchartered territory and discovering narrative forms capable of relating this adventure as it unfolds.[7]

Dingdingdong was founded around the traumatic experience of how Alice Rivière (the written persona of Emilie Hermant) gained knowledge, through predictive testing, of having the genetic status of being a gene carrier for Huntington's. *Dingdingdong* focused initially on the issue of presymptomatic diagnosis, although the collaborative work and website is also dedicated to coproducing knowledge regarding the question of how people live with Huntington's, with knowledge and with symptoms, knowledge of symptoms, and symptoms of knowledge.

The *Dingdingdong Manifesto* was published in 2013 and, in addition to being an apposite and moving testimony of diagnosis, interconnects a number of themes and questions that are pertinent for those confronted with the reality of ALS, even though the specificity of the diagnosis and test is distinct.

Unlike Huntington's, there is no test for ALS. It is a clinical diagnosis founded on exclusion. This is frequently considered a problem. It can take time to be sure. From first signs that begin to worry an individual to a diagnosis, it can take up to a year or sometimes more. What the *Dingdingdong Manifesto* (2013) and the recent book by Katrin Solhdju, *Testing Knowledge: Toward an Ecology of Diagnosis* (2021), show, however, is that knowledge, in itself, is not connected to any virtue other than itself. To know is one thing. What one can then do with that knowledge is another. Knowing in and of itself may be a virtue, but if it is one, its only virtue is that one knows. Its relation to any others or to other vices is an open question. Solhdju and Alice Rivière (author of the *Manifesto*) ask how knowledge can be connected to—as well as bracketed, reformulated, transformed, and used to think about, talk about, and narrate—a life lived with a diagnosis.

The diagnosis is particular and shares only a little with ALS. Huntington's is an autosomal dominant, monogenic disease with full penetrance. If a person has a parent with the illness, it means that a parent has a copy of the single gene that causes the illness, which is on the short arm of chromosome 4. The gene in question, which was named *Huntingtin*, contains an area of DNA where the same three bases are repeated multiple times, in this case a cytosine, adenine, guanine (CAG) nucleotide triplet. When this CAG triplet occurs in over forty repeats, the penetrance is 100 percent, meaning the person with the gene will develop the illness. A child of one parent with the gene will therefore have a 50 percent chance of having inherited it, increasing to a 75 percent chance if both parents have the gene.

There is an inherited form of ALS, but it is highly uncommon. I touch on it only in passing in this book. What the *Manifesto*, as well as the work of *Dingdingdong*, provides for those of us thinking about other neurological diseases is how to bring together, if at all, knowledge, countenance, and ways of talking and writing, speculating, and acting in relation to a diagnosis, one that, as it stands today, from a medical point of view, has no curative response. The challenge laid down by *Dingdingdong* is how, with the support of a novel institution dedicated to coproducing new forms of knowledge, to provide new ways of responding to such a diagnosis.

For my purposes, I underscore two points raised by Alice Rivière in the *Manifesto*: her observation of what she calls the "anybodyfication" (*quiconquisation*) of the medical apparatus that configures knowledge of a genetic status with a diagnosis foretold, since technically it is not a diagnosis as there are not yet symptoms. As I understand it, the work of those involved in coproducing knowledge within *Dingdingdong* is to contest the anybodyfication of the medical apparatus. The means of doing so is the second point I want to underscore: drawing on the work of the American philosopher William James (1842–1910), Rivière writes of distinguishing between "live" and "dead" propositions to belief: with dead propositions being those in which one is treated as already dead and yet (paradoxically) also expected to show "good behavior," to listen to the genetic counselor, to not want to end one's life, to be sad and angry but not too sad or angry, especially not against the medical apparatus that offered this possibility of knowing. One could say, following Canguilhem, for the sick person to not seek to impose their own, new norms of what it could signify to live with illness.

These two points are important for what follows. I too saw a form of clinical *bodyfication*, not *anybodyfication* but rather a *this-body-fication*, in which the question of to *whom this*-body belongs, a question of identity, a question of the subject, was left open, albeit bracketed. This seems to be a difference with the *any*-bodyfication Rivière writes of, which would seem to lead to a "*nobody*-fication" or perhaps, more specifically, a *bodily-nobodyfication*. Second, there is a shared question of the prefiguration of suffering: to know, or to have a sense of knowing, or thinking one knows what is to come. With Huntington's, however, it is a presymptomatic prefiguration, which makes a difference. The shared question, between Huntington's and ALS, is how to make something "living" out of the test or out of the diagnosis, of leaving open the question of how to live a diagnosis that takes the form of a prediction.

Lastly, I have taken note of several medical anthropological studies that have inquired into Parkinson's disease (*paralysis agitans*). Parkinson's is a neurological disorder caused by degenerative disease of the basal ganglia, associated with rigidity, tremor, poverty of movement, odd posture, and peculiar acceleration of gait. Unlike ALS, a range of treatments have been developed that have greatly improved life expectancy and symptom management, such as levodopa and the use of dopamine agonists and monoamine oxidase-B inhibitors, although the side effects and the lack of long-term sustainability of their use mean that there are trade-offs in symptom management. Deep brain stimulation has also been developed to manage symptoms.

In the anthropological literature, the work of two researchers stands out, Samantha Solimeo and Narelle Warren. Solimeo took up the experience of rural Americans with Parkinson's, considering it a "condition" and not a "disease." She describes how her informants unknotted the role of the "sick" person, an approach that thus simultaneously draws on functionalist sociological studies of illness in the lineage of Talcott Parsons and shows a variant with respect to such a functionalist view. Rather than considering themselves "sick," Solimeo shows how at very specific moments, individuals make evaluations and distinctions between "aging" and the effects of Parkinson's as a specific condition. Warren's research has taken up several different approaches, one of which is very much in line with Solimeo's focus on the "everyday" experience, particularly the idiopathic and uncertain character of Parkinson's. Uncertainty here refers to the unpredictability of day-to-day "experience," a term by which Warren and her coauthor Darshini Ayton point to the variability of symptoms. The authors write of how the "embodied experience of Parkinson's forces a daily reconciliation of the who will I be with how do I feel and what can I do,"[8] which appears, like Solimeo's account, to blur the lines between the specificity of having a disease and the more general phenomenon of being alive and asking oneself questions about who and how one is.

Myopathies, Huntington's, and Parkinson's have been taken up as objects of study in the social sciences, and the work on these illnesses provides resources and tools to think with and about the specificity of ALS: patient participation in research and the reframing of research agendas; questions of identity and of the relation to knowledge, to genetic testing, and to futures foretold; the specificity of language use in neurodegenerative illness; and questions about how degeneration links to conceptions of aging. My own approach underscores the importance of what can be called, in a broad sense, "working-through" ALS, for patients, families, friends, and medical professionals, in relation to medical and scientific knowledge, clinical apparatuses, and the open question of how to orient the singularity of a life to this illness. The "work" of working-through is not the same for each, and each singular existence countenances it or endeavors to forge a countenance, as they can or as they do. Despite this singularity, and also because of that singularity, a question, I will contend, is shared: how to countenance the losses linked to this particular illness.

The Necessity of History

Fieldwork, conducted from August 2019–March 2020, was a necessary but not sufficient means of knowing something about what people are confronted with when they are confronted with ALS. To assemble and arrange the elements in relation to which and through which different people—people with ALS, their families and friends, neurologists and other medical specialists—encounter this illness, today, to understand the range of practices, forms of knowledge, and ways of being that give shape to how people encounter this illness, as an object, it was necessary to engage in historical work with respect to two key moments: 1875 and 1975. These two dates are obligatory reference points in how ALS became an object of thought and how it became problematized in specific ways.

Methodologically, I began with fieldwork in the present, at the ALS clinic. As I endeavored to grasp the state of current knowledge about the illness, in order to understand contemporary neurological knowledge, I was obliged to retrace the emergence of the disease category. Hence, I started from the moment at which the illness was first conceptualized as a disease entity, by Jean-Martin Charcot in 1875, and then moved backward to the early nineteenth century, taking Charles Bell's *Idea of a New Anatomy of the Brain* (1811) as my starting point, to then investigate the sequence of neurological writings about the nervous system that constituted available medical knowledge about motor issues, leading up to 1875, and then after this key date at which the disease category was named, to continue on from 1875 to the contemporary, asking what has changed in the available medical knowledge about the illness. My way of proceeding could broadly fit into what Hans-Jörg Rheinberger has named as "historical epistemology."[9]

To put it very briefly, since this will be described at length over the course of the book, the first date, 1875, is the moment at which a form of anatomo-physical knowledge of the illness emerged, knowledge that has been problematized since 1890 with respect to two key indeterminations: (1) the correlation between cognitive and motor symptoms in patients with ALS (since the late nineteenth century) and (2) the molecular–causal pathway (since the late twentieth century).

The year 1875 is when Charcot made public his nosological work establishing the diagnosis of ALS, linking surface signs and symptoms with a neurophysiological and pathological account of the corresponding sites of degeneration. Despite all of the advances in medicine, physiology, and molecular biology, at the time of writing in 2021, biomedical understanding of the causes of the illness, like most neurological illnesses, is scant further advanced, providing both a sense of certitude and a range of uncertainties.

This point is hard to overstate relative to the core preoccupation of this book: unlike other objects of inquiry in medical anthropology or the medical humanities, the fact that this is an illness that is still universally fatal, with very little change in terms of prognosis, which at the same time is an object of inquiry, inquiry circling around the holes in our neurological knowledge, means that it is a countercase and counternarrative to those that often interest anthropologists, which is to say, emerging knowledge of disease (e.g., the story and history of COVID-19), the development of new treatments, equitable access to those treatments, or questions about how "cure" is linked to care.[10] This is not to say that there has been "no" new knowledge or "no" new treatments, and as we will see at the very end of the book, with respect to those few clinical trials in progress, patients with ALS, like other patient groups, have been advocating for things like "expanded access," which is the use of an unapproved drug in a clinical trial by those who were excluded or unable to enroll in the trial.[11] It is to say, rather, that the historical backdrop against which contemporary experience plays out is crucial to understand the viscosity and density of the situation that those confronted with ALS as an object of experience must face. Unlike inquiries into AIDS, cancer care, or tuberculosis, the anthropologist cannot take an event, the "war on cancer," new therapies, or the twenty-year period of "political work" that defined the public policy, ethical, economic, and public health questions linked to the AIDS epidemic, globally, as an object of attention. In a certain sense, all those concerned by ALS are waiting, hence hoping—hoping for an event that will disrupt the viscosity in the knowledge and care that has emerged over the past one hundred and fifty years.

Such viscosity notwithstanding, what is more variable, with a larger degree of freedom, however, is the attitude a person takes toward this illness, given the state of affairs in terms of knowledge and given the apparatuses of medical care available. It is on this point that the second date, 1975, is crucial and gives a specific shape to how ALS can appear as an object of consideration and as a problem to be confronted, for patients, families, and health workers: the question of medical attitude toward the illness, and those with this illness, was raised in 1975 in practical terms, meaning, how should physicians, nurses, patients, and family members orient themselves both to the available knowledge of the illness and to the bodily reality of this illness?

Part 1
KNOWLEDGE

Today, two decades into the twenty-first century, it has become a commonplace of medical history, following the foundational work of historian and philosopher Michel Foucault (1926–1984), to consider the nineteenth century as the turning point at which the "medical gaze" (*le regard médical*) was institutionalized.[1] By way of this term, a transformation in medical perception was posited and tracked over the course of the nineteenth century: "The presence of disease in the body, with its tensions and burnings, the silent world of the entrails, the whole dark underside of the body lined with endless unseeing dreams, are challenged as to their objectivity by the reductive discourse of the doctor, as well as established as multiple objects meeting his positive gaze."[2] The elegant and lucid historical diagnosis expounded by Foucault in his 1966 *The Birth of the Clinic* remains, in its broad contours, a trenchant account of how sight and knowledge were configured, in relation to the space of the body, over the course of the nineteenth century, notwithstanding efforts of medical historians, among them notably Roy Porter, to bracket Foucault's overarching account of the emergence of the medical gaze, in favor of "the patient's view," a view that David Armstrong nevertheless has shown is not mutually exclusive to its being constituted by such a gaze.[3]

The two chapters that follow, which both concern forms of medical knowledge about ALS, could be understood as constituting merely a case in point of the broader argument, already so well known, applied to neurology: the anatomo-clinical method, through which such a gaze was operationalized, rendered possible a configuration of surface signs with anatomic sites in the field of neurology, signs later reconfigured and rendered problematic by the emergence of molecular knowledge of the disease.[4] This is not my aim. Or rather, it is not my ultimate aim.

Such a case in point is rather the necessary legwork, propaedeutic to the endeavor of trying to grasp a problem, namely: given the anatomo-clinical knowledge that has come to be established, over 150 years (1870–2020), about motor neuron diseases and knowledge of illnesses that are still to this day incurable, and given the confusion, indetermination, and the expectations of—and demands for—progress, stemming from ever increasing molecular knowledge of these illnesses, developed in the first two decades of the twenty-first century, how does a person live with this knowledge, expectation of progress, and disappointment with the lack of progress?

In the case of ALS, an illness for which neurologists still do not have molecular tests to aid with diagnosis or significant therapies, clinical knowledge of the illness is confirmed or disconfirmed in the progression of the disease: the patient's experience of something being wrong may lead to a clinical diagnosis, albeit without clear knowledge of the disease mechanism in biological terms, and the diagnosis is confirmed or disconfirmed in experience.

The question that follows for the person living with the illness, and with that diagnosis, is how to give form to that knowledge, if at all, and more important, how to give form to a life with that knowledge—namely, how to conduct one's life, both with the experience of illness and with a certain awareness and knowledge about that illness and that experience.

Such an indetermination can only be answered by hearing from those who live with such illness. Nevertheless, it is crucial to understand that those with illness and those who are trying to care for them are living not only in relation to an experience of symptoms but also in relation to knowledge—namely, what can be known about that illness, as well as in relation to an understanding of illness, which is to say, an illness that becomes theirs (through experience).

A second commonplace, then, is in order and this time from medical anthropology—the proposition that the task of thinking about illness is to reconnect knowledge of pathology with the normativity of the subject who endeavors to live with it and in relation to it.

What I seek to trace here in part 1 of this book is how knowledge of ALS was first produced and how it has, to a large degree, become a stabilized diagnosis, which admits of only limited uncertainty. That is, limited uncertainty once the diagnosis is given. And so, given its relative certitude and its lack of treatment, which is to say treatments that can halt or reverse the illness, unlike in some other medical domains, my task is to ask how the illness challenges patients, families, caregivers, and medical staff to live and work and care with and in relation to knowledge of this disease.

In chapter 1, I narrate the emergence of neurological knowledge of the illness by starting from a moment when there was no such thing as ALS, a known diagnostic entity (i.e., prior to 1875). The chapter opens with a specific moment when the neurological symptoms of the illness could nevertheless be described, circa 1836, thanks to the then available understanding (since roughly 1811) of the separation and function of sensory and motor neurological pathways. I seek subsequently to trace the development of neurological knowledge through to the achievement of a named illness (Charcot's disease/motor neuron diseases/amyotrophic lateral sclerosis) and then move forward to a clinical moment in the present, in which a patient is suspected of having the illness, thus configuring three moments circa 1836, circa 1880, and 2019.

My objective, in configuring these historical moments, the forms of knowledge mobilized, and the norms of practice displayed, is not to say that nothing has changed since the high point of the late nineteenth century. What I want to explore is how clinical knowledge of the illness, as an arrangement of signs, has not significantly changed, such that the question of the viscosity of knowledge of ALS may then subsequently be linked to the question of significance of this arrangement of signs: how to live with knowledge of the illness (i.e., in relation to that arrangement).

A second chapter then takes up an indetermination that ruffles the sense of certitude outlined in chapter 1; it is not a thwarting of the diagnosis per se but rather of the nosological status of "the" disease being diagnosed, which ultimately, despite the sense of certitude that still accompanies the diagnosis, nevertheless indexes a syndrome as well as an anatomopathologically localizable disease entity. Very specifically, an issue that has accompanied, not to say haunted, knowledge of ALS is the co-occurrence in disease progression of different kinds of dementias or cognitive problems along with motor neuron degeneration.

Is it mere coincidence? Or does the overlap between ALS and cognitive issues, broadly considered, tell us something more fundamental about this neurodegenerative illness, knowledge of which could undermine the notion that this supposedly purely neuromuscular degeneration can be separated from neuropsychiatric issues? This concern has subtended knowledge of ALS as a disease entity since the 1890s.

To rephrase the question: Given the analytic sense of certitude that came with the anatomopathological method in the 1870s, which identified ALS as a distinct disease category, how is the diagnostic co-occurrence of motor neuron and cognitive degeneration, known by way of clinical symptoms, anatomical signs, and molecular biological traces, arranged and understood to be, or not as the case may be, part of *a* disease?

Whereas in the nineteenth century, anatomopathology was the decisive tool for knowing ALS, today, the molecular biological underpinnings of the various clinical signs, along with neuroimaging and neuropathological findings, are the means through which hypotheses are made about the possibility that a variety of neurodegenerative illnesses stem from common underlying disease processes. The indetermination and challenge is then to integrate the clinical, pathological, and molecular understandings of the syndrome of ALS, so as to give a form to a possible knowledge—an integration that is, however, still lacking.

THE EMERGENCE OF A DIAGNOSTIC CERTITUDE

An undated case note, communicated to the Scottish surgeon, neurologist, and anatomist Sir Charles Bell (1774–1842) by a Mr. Budd, was published by Bell in 1836 in an expanded third edition of his *The Nervous System of the Human Body*, including an "appendix of cases" with this particular description exemplifying "Loss of Motion, Sensation Remaining".[1]

> A labourer's wife, aet. [aged] 41, was seized, while apparently in good health, first with weakness of the left foot, and, in five weeks afterwards, with weakness of the right foot. This did not prevent her, for some time, from walking with assistance, but gradually she was altogether deprived of motion in her legs, and was confined to bed. It was remarkable that she experienced no diminution of the sensibility of the skin of the affected parts. Being unable to shift her position in bed, she suffered very much from the pressure against the points of bone in lying; and to get relief, she was obliged to keep one of her children always beside her to change her position. She wakened her child frequently in the night, to obtain her assistance in turning herself round. A fleabite distressed her, yet she could not move to scratch herself! A year after the commencement of the complaint, the weakness extended to the arms, and she began to experience difficulty in her breathing. The accessory muscles of respiration in the neck and chest were then seen to act with remarkable force. Her general health had been good until the paralysis reached the superior extremities, when she gradually got worse, suffering

mostly from difficulty of respiration, and died in six weeks. No examination of the body could be obtained.[2]

The case was presented without commentary: we know nothing of where she lived and died, who she was, and how the physician knew her, and we know nothing of what Mr. Budd thought of the illness, other than the fact that a brief description warranted being sent to the most well-known neurologist in Great Britain.

The description of the patient's affliction, as well as the relative ignorance of its characteristics, was narrated by Budd in a mixed genre, characterized by a mood somewhere between medical report and village news, perhaps indicating how knowledge of the case was transmitted. Within Bell's appendix, the case served to underscore, in simple terms, what had become, by then, a medical commonplace: by the 1830s, it had become part of medical knowledge that there is an anatomical separation of motor and sensory function, by way of distinct roots, and it was known to observers by this time that neurological illness could affect one function while sparing the other.

A quarter century earlier, in 1811, Bell had published his *Idea of a New Anatomy of the Brain*, some of the core ideas for which had been outlined in exchanges of letters with his brother George Joseph Bell, including the conception of an anatomical division between sensory and motor nerves. With a sense of the historical magnitude of the discoveries he was laying out in *Anatomy of the Brain*, he summarized, for his brother's benefit, his idea that parts of the brain were distinct in function: "It occurred to me that there were four grand divisions of the brain, so were there four grand divisions of the spinal marrow; first, a lateral division, then a division into the back and forepart. Next, it occurred to me that all the spinal nerves had within the sheath of the spinal marrow two roots—one from the back part, another from before. Whenever this occurred to me I thought that I had obtained a method of inquiry into the function of the parts of the brain."[3] What became known as the "the priority dispute" over the discovery of the roots of motor and sensory nerves is well known, with Bell sharing in the discovery with François Magendie (1783–1855).[4] The Bell–Magendie law, as it was subsequently named, established that the anterior spinal nerve roots contain only motor fibers and posterior roots only sensory fibers, and moreover, that nerve impulses are conducted in only one direction, in each set of fibers.

The clinical picture described by Budd, of motor degeneration with sensory function intact, left open, however, the question of both the etiology of such motor path illness and the link between the clinical and pathological understanding of the illness. No comment as to the nature of the paralysis and weakness was made in 1836, or any comment as to the manner in which the illness came on, its steady course, and the possible interventions that were made, if any.

A Sense of Certitude

Half a century later: February 28, 1888, Jean-Martin Charcot (1825–1893) conducted his (even at the time) famous Tuesday lesson at the Pitié-Salpêtrière hospital in Paris.[5] He would have been briefed on the patient, but part of the performance, and of the spectacle, was for the auditors to see in practice the clinical diagnosis, with its moments of hesitation, reflection, and brilliant demonstration of certitude.[6] The following narrative is curated from a published translated transcription of a public diagnosis by Charcot.[7]

A fifty-seven-year-old man and his son are presented to him. The patient is described as holding a handkerchief over his mouth. Charcot asks the audience to note the detail of the handkerchief, its purpose being to catch the patient's drooling spittle, which his son confirms occurs continuously. It is especially problematic when eating. Charcot asks how long it takes for his father to eat his meals. Although he has good appetite, it takes him over an hour, the son explains. Charcot asks him to describe the consistency of the meals that his father eats: "His meat is cut into tiny slivers because he cannot chew well." He then asks what happens with fluids: "Fluids go down the wrong way and he chokes." As to whether these problems came on suddenly or progressively, he explains that his father's problems emerged slowly, and when asked to be more specific, he describes how his father began speaking abnormally, about fourteen months previously, and then continued to deteriorate "to the point where now he cannot speak at all."

"Is his memory intact?" Charcot asks. Yes. Turning his attention directly to the patient, Charcot asks whether he can write, and his son replies on his father's behalf, saying that he writes quite well. This will be a first crucial turning point in the diagnosis. Turning his attention to the audience, Charcot reiterates the state of affairs: "He maintains his ability to write in the face of absolutely no speech."

The loss of speech could suggest a diagnosis of aphasia, and Charcot then specifies that this could be either (a transcortical) motor aphasia or Broca's aphasia (a type of aphasia characterized by partial loss of the ability to produce language). He rules out these options based on the fact that "it is rare, in fact absolutely exceptional to see a true aphasic patient of this sort write with facility."

Charcot breaks the suspense and connects an identification of the speech pathology to a possible diagnosis: "In fact, we are faced with a case of bulbar palsy. You know that in my Friday lecture, we discussed the topic, specifically its relation to amyotrophic lateral sclerosis. The case before us will allow us today to take that information and apply it clinically. I am going to try to show you the necessary steps to arrive at a proper diagnosis and prognosis." The case before the audience, Charcot recapitulates, conforms to the description by Duchenne de Boulogne of glossolabial–laryngeal paralysis, developing slowly and progressing.[8] Charcot asks the patient to open his mouth partly: "With his left hand he [Charcot] holds the blade of a paper opener against the front of the patient's lower teeth and presses firmly, while with his right hand he taps the paper opener with a Skoda hammer":

> I am working on some research involving jaw reflexes. You see how each time I hit the jaw, the lower jaw jumps with a quick jerk. This means that the reflex we are examining is accentuated. Can we draw any conclusions from such an observation? Indeed. Up to this point, I have remained a bit reserved in my evaluation of this case. All we could say is, "glossolabial-laryngeal paralysis." But this term, in fact, does not describe a single disease, for there are several categories. With all due respect to Duchenne de Boulogne, this is a syndrome [glossolabial–laryngeal paralysis], but not a diagnosis.
>
> Now with the information provided by the jaw jerk, we can say much more and declare that in all probability, the progressive bulbar palsy in this case belongs to the subtype known as amyotrophic lateral sclerosis with apparent sparing so far of the extremities. I say "in all probability" and cannot be more certain because it could be that the responsible lesions, if situated in selected regions of both hemispheres so as to interrupt the cortical bulbar fibers (that is, cortical-lingual, cortical-glossal, etc.) could produce this same exaggerated jaw jerk, along with the bulbar syndrome. This is called pseudobulbar palsy. But this latter condition proceeds by discrete episodes of apoplectic attacks, whereas in today's case, the progression, as far as we have monitored it, is essentially slow and continual. We are dealing therefore with amyotrophic lateral sclerosis, which instead of starting in the upper and lower extremities, as is the usual pattern with only very late bulbar involvement, has started the other way around. This is my diagnosis, and in all likelihood it will be confirmed by the rest of the examination.

Charcot then adds considerations of anatomopathology: "If we observe in the extremities paresis and tendon reflex exaggeration, it would be reasonable to conclude that these signs relate to lateral column involvement, whereas amyotrophy and fasciculations indicate the involvement of the anterior horn cell."[9] At this stage, Charcot has in effect summarized the state of knowledge about amyotrophic lateral sclerosis at that time, in 1888.

La sclérose latérale amyotrophique (amyotrophic lateral sclerosis, ALS): the name given by Charcot to an illness that combines signs of lesion in the lateral corticospinal tract, signs of paresis and hyperreflexivity, and the telltale signs of muscle wasting typical of degeneration of the anterior horn cells of the gray matter in the spinal column.

Charcot proposed, in the lesson cited above, a differential diagnosis of Broca's or motor aphasia.[10] He gave his reasons for considering this a clear case of bulbar palsy, an indication of a possible sign of amyotrophic lateral sclerosis, seemingly confirmed by the exaggerated jaw reflex, which, due to the steady progression of the illness, indicates ALS rather than pseudobulbar palsy.

In Charcot's view, which was first published in 1875, when motor degeneration exhibits both kinds of signs, both spasticity and muscle wasting, then the amyotrophy (muscle wasting) is consequent to, and follows on from, the sclerosis of the lateral columns, which is exhibited by signs of spastic tone—hence, in the terminology invented by Charcot, "amyotrophic" is the qualifying term of the main neurological issue of "lateral sclerosis."

The Tuesday patient was subsequently asked to undress and whether he could dress himself, to which the response was negative. The examination of his lower extremities indicated a compromised gait, weakness due to spasticity, and emaciated thighs, although sensation was determined to be intact, in keeping with a suspicion of a pure motor degeneration. Charcot concluded with assuredness:

> Amyotrophic lateral sclerosis with bulbar onset. The diagnosis in such a case carries with it, and note this well, a sense of certitude, one can say of absolute precision, showing thus to what point neuropathology has become her own mistress in certain areas.
>
> (*To the patient*) My friend, you can leave the room now and you will be told in a minute what you can do in order to get well. (*The patient leaves*).
>
> Now, gentlemen, that the patient is no longer here, we can and must speak amongst ourselves in total frankness. The prognosis is deplorable; alas, he is a lost soul, and it is only a question of time.
>
> No matter what is done, the bulbar dysfunction will progress relentlessly. Feeding will become more and more difficult. The pulse will rise in the final phase, signaling the end, and respiratory compromise will set in. It is sad to say, but it is true.
>
> . . . However, for the doctor, whether it is sad or not is not the issue; truth is the issue. Let the patient live in illusion to the end, that is fine; it is humane and the best way. But the doctor, is it his role to do the same? We are sometimes reproached for conducting incessant studies on the major neurologic diseases, which have, up to now, mostly been

incurable. What use is it? It has almost come to the point where people have questioned whether this is really medicine.[11]

ALS Clinic

September 25, 2019, and it is 131 years after the scene at the Salpêtrière: the Wednesday clinic at the hospital. It's 8 A.M. People are coming into clinic, winding their way through the corridors that snake around to a large waiting room and then on into cramped consulting rooms that back on to an office area. That morning I found James, the registered dietician at the board, a white board located on the eastern half of this space that twice a week receives patients.

The board indicates, in rows, the initials of the patients who have been checked in. Patients are divided broadly into two sessions, morning and afternoon, with usually around six in each session. The board is also divided into columns, for the different specialists that make up this multidisciplinary team: physical therapy (PT), occupational therapy (OT), speech and language pathology (SLP), the registered dietician ("the dietician"), respiratory therapy ("respiratory"), the social worker from the ALS Association, the research coordinator, and, of course, the neurologist as well as a resident in neurology and possibly a fellow or a student. Patients wait in the atrium until roomed and then are seen one by one in a not necessarily preplanned but still coordinated manner by the different specialties, depending on the wants and needs of the patients and families.

A team meeting usually starts off the day in which the team reviews the patients' charts, going through the list according to appointment time, with the aim being to refresh everyone's memory as to who the patient is and to read through any particular needs or comments that either the team noted from a previous visit or exchanges with the patient leading up to the visit or from the clinic nurse's notes following the previsit telephone consultations that the clinic nurse conducts.

These consultations are used to find out any particular issues the patient may have, and importantly, it is when the nurse fills out a "functional rating scale" (FRS) for the patient. The FRS is a set of twelve questions that are scored 0 to 4, with 0 indicating "no function" and 4 indicating "full function" for the following items: speech, salivation, swallowing, handwriting, cutting food/using utensils, dressing/hygiene, turning in bed, walking, climbing stairs, difficulty breathing (dyspnea), and difficulty breathing while lying flat (orthopnea).

On this particular day, as I walked in, I was directed away from chart review.

I Hope It Is Not ALS

"Good morning." James turned to me and suggested straightaway that I follow a neurology resident, Lilith. She'll be meeting a new patient. "He's really far along, very bulbar, doesn't have a diagnosis but it looks really bad." James, more than others in the team, expresses his thoughts about diagnosis, whether it looks likely or probable, whether he'd be surprised if it wasn't, and so on. He has been with the center for almost a decade, previously having worked at another ALS clinic. Lilith knows how the team works, he told me, since she was a research coordinator here before going to medical school. She'll be seeing the new patient this morning, a Mr. Bay, so I could go in with her, he told me. He went to check if it would be okay. James introduced us and explained why I was there at the clinic. We went to the waiting room.

Mr. Bay walked with some difficulty. We went into the small windowless room. "He's claustrophobic," Mrs. Bay told me. Mr. Bay explained that he is quite difficult to understand, pointing to his throat, and then at his wife. She's his interpreter. For the most part, I missed quite a bit of what he said, but I came to realize that the information that the resident needed, at least in terms of medical history, is relatively simple and discernable, and the nuances of his life and his story, while important for him, are not crucial to knowing the truth of his illness. The illness, to a large degree, speaks for itself.

"You have an EMG [electromyography] scheduled at one. Dr. Blumen will be in charge, and she will come in to see you later, and we'll figure out who else in the team it would be good to see." Mr. Bay said that it sounds good. Lilith continued, "So I was reading about how all of this started. Your first symptoms were slurred speech a year ago. Nothing before that?" No. "What next?" His neck. He had trouble holding up his head. Muscle weakness. "When did that start?" In April. "Difficulty swallowing?" Yes. He went to a doctor. He was sent to a swallow specialist, Mrs. Bay specified. "I see in your file that the exam showed some food and fluid going down the wrong tube. It looks like ENT diagnosed right vocal cord paralysis. You were sent for an MRI of the soft tissue of the neck. Eating?" It's difficult, Mr. Bay said. "Change in consistency?" He told the doctor he had lost 75 lbs. since April. "Saliva?" Yes, it's like phlegm sticking to the vocal cords, he explained. "Drooling?" A little. "Weakness in arms and legs?" The left side, his arm, there's no muscle left. The resident repeats what she understood. "You noticed a decrease in muscle size everywhere, and when did the left arm start to feel weak?" In April as well.

"Which hand do you write with?" The left. "How do you write?" Mr. Bay demonstrates, pretending to write in the air, using his right hand to hold his left hand at its base. "Is your handwriting legible or is it getting sloppier?" It's getting sloppier, Mr. Bay smiled. I endeavored to restrain the lugubriousness that swelled inside me. "Can you feed yourself and dress yourself?" He can hold a knife, but it has to be very sharp. Dressing himself, sometimes it's the buttons that are difficult, pants or shirt buttons. "Do you still have the problem with your neck, holding your head up?" Yes. "Pain?" Yes, and weakness, he says. "Trouble turning over in bed?" He says he just sleeps on one side. Mrs. Bay intervenes to tell Mr. Bay that the doctor is asking if he can't turn over at night. Mr. Bay ignores his wife.

"Walking?" He says he stumbles here and there and tells Lilith that he was a golfer in the '70s. Lilith didn't appear to have understood what he had said, smiled, nodded her head, and turned her gaze back to her computer. I thought I saw a brief look of disappointment on his face when she didn't ask him about it. I considered repeating what he had said, but then thought better of it. "Stairs?" Stairs are okay, with a handrail. His shortness of breath started with the throat issues.

"Everything started going to pot in April," Mrs. Bay clarified.

"Do you notice twitching?" No. Mrs. Bay says that he doesn't feel them, but she can feel them, when they're in bed. Lilith looks at his arms; she thinks she can see some twitches, and then says no, that maybe it was just his pulse. "Do you ever find yourself laughing or crying inappropriately?" No. He says that his wife makes him laugh, pointing at his wife. "So it's always appropriate." Perhaps because it's on the subject of his emotions, he tells Lilith that he plays golf in his head to get to sleep. He's had anxiety for a long time, he says.

"Have you noticed any cognitive problems? No trouble with memory?" Lilith asks. Mrs. Bay looks at me and says that "maybe it's a male thing, I have to repeat myself." Lilith clarifies her question by asking Mr. Bay whether he has any difficulty finding words. No. "I'm better at *Jeopardy* than her!" Lilith asks if there are any dementia or cognitive problems in the family. "My father was an alcoholic. My brother had a gambling problem and committed suicide: one day he got a big debt and that was it." Lilith asks if it was a sudden change, in adulthood. "No, he inherited from my dad." Lilith is searching for clues as to whether there is a family history that could indicate frontotemporal dementia, a non-Alzheimer's type of dementia characterized by behavioral and affective problems.[12]

"Are your muscles hard to move?" He doesn't have any, he tells Lilith. "The primary [primary care physician] doesn't think it's anything bad," Mrs. Bay says. She goes on to explain, with a good deal of frustration, that everything, every step of the way, they had to ask for—to see the swallow specialist, to see a pulmonary specialist, to get an appointment with a neurologist. Lilith says that they've been great advocates. "The primary wanted to send him to a psychiatrist!" Mrs. Bay exclaims, exasperated, and shaking her head.

"I hope it's not ALS," Mr. Bay says. "I hope that the weakness is coming from my neck."

"I'm going to examine you now: can you tell me today's date?" 9-25-19. She points to her watch and asks him what it is. "A fancy one, nicer than mine," he says, lifting up his wrist. The resident did not ask him to say the word "watch." "This part of the hand?" He tells her that they're knuckles. She tests his eye movement and asks him to push air into his cheeks and to show her his teeth. Lilith touches both sides of his face, at the top, middle, and bottom: "Does it feel the same on both sides?" Yes. She asks him to show her his tongue. "You don't want to see his tongue!" Mrs. Bay interjects.

"I see what you mean about muscle loss in the hands." Lilith took a pocket light and began to search for fasciculation and then felt for tone.

"May I interrupt? Did you notice his crooked shoulders?" Mrs. Bay asked. "PT [physical therapy] is trying to get him to drop them down but it's no use. It's been going on for a few months."

"Any numbness?" Just when he's driving. Lilith takes out her reflex hammer: "Can you feel this buzzing?" Yes. "Toes?" He feels pressure but no buzzing. She checks his reflexes. Taps his knees, his arms, his heels. "I'm going to check the reflex in your jaw as well"; she repeats what she is about to do, explaining that it may feel a little odd, and she taps him. Then, she asks him to walk outside in the corridor.

"He's trying to impress her," Mrs. Bay says to me. She calls out down the hall after him: "Where do you normally put your hand, Barney!??" Mr. Bay switches its position, from having his hands at his side to placing his right hand over his right hip and thigh. "I put it here," he says with a grin, "to make me more stable." We went back into the exam room. Lilith finishes writing some notes and then tells the couple that some other people will be in to see them and that he has the EMG at one. We leave the room and walk over to the board.

James came over to see Lilith while she was writing up Mr. Bay's chart. "Maybe only lower motor neuron, as it is mainly muscle wasting and reduced tone," she said. "But the reflexes were brisk. Jaw jerk, I didn't get too much of a response. He's lost 75 lbs. since April." She tells James that he can go in to see him. Lilith then went over to the computer and signaled for me to come and see. "The MRI they did outside of the hospital, at some other provider, was for soft tissue of the neck, which is irrelevant," she said, "but the images do show the spinal column." She flicked through the images and found what she was looking for: images of the cervical vertebrae. "If it were C spine disease, we would see compressions resulting in patches without CFS [cerebrospinal fluid]." She flicks through the vertebrae, the central column of the spine surrounded by a ring of white, the fluid. On one image, it looks a little thinner but is still present, forming a ring. "C spine disease can mimic ALS, but if it's C spine it's below the neck, and he has tongue fasciculation. So, he has diffuse atrophy, diffuse hyper-reflexia, and fasciculation in the tongue. How many regions does it need to be? Three? I should know this," she said. The El Escorial criteria require three regions with upper and lower motor neuron signs for a "definite" diagnosis. Lilith checked the hospital's *Up to Date* database. "So, three regions (cervical, thoracic, and lumbosacral), upper and lower, with the upper sign being brisk reflexes."

Names and Locations, 1840–1899: A Disease of the Motor Neurons, Upper and Lower

While the tools had changed, the essential knowledge enacted by Lilith had not changed since the diagnostic performance by Charcot in 1888. Although it is true that the imaging results were important for clarity over the differential diagnosis, the question (how to explain Mr. Bay's clinical tableau) and the methods (physical exam and questioning) were in keeping with the scene from the late nineteenth century. The half-century leading up to Charcot's diagnosis saw the emergence of a very specific shift in how knowledge of pathology was connected to disease classification, in the living, suffering patient, a shift that made possible the naming of this disease, consequent to the specification of anatomic lesions that produce the clinical tableau. The vague description of "weakness"—a constant in our case histories from 1836 to 2019—was anatomically localized in the lateral columns and in the anterior horn of the gray matter. The lesions located in these two distinct sites were known by way of distinct signs: atrophy and spasticity. By the time of the "Tuesday lesson," Charcot was supremely confident in the state of neurological knowledge about this illness. As he put it, "The diagnosis as well as the anatomy and physiology of the condition amyotrophic lateral sclerosis is one of the most completely understood conditions in the realm of clinical neurology."[13] In a very specific sense, Charcot was not wrong: the phenotype of the clinical presentation, heterogeneous though it may well be—in two of the cases above, the presentation is a less common form of "bulbar onset"—is highly recognizable: one of the crowning achievements of nineteenth-century neurology was to be able to correlate clinical signs to lesions in the spine and brain, and the nature of those lesions was increasingly specified.

Charcot's confidence was vindicated as neurology discovered its core unit of concern. Just a short time after the clinical encounter of 1888, as a Parisian winter turned to a Spanish summer, Santiago Ramón y Cajal (1852–1934) showed definitively that nerve cells were not continuous in the brain of birds, and in 1891, the anatomist Heinrich Wilhelm Gottfried von Waldeyer-Hartz (1836–1921) proposed the term "neuron" to identify this fundamental neurological object. It would take just a few years for his term to be used with facility in neurological discourse. In 1895, Sanger Brown (1852–1928) gave a talk on "The Neuron in Medicine," reprinted in the *Journal of the American Medical Association*, ebullient about the state of neurological knowledge and the change in the neurological training of students since the late 1880s. Thanks to the term "neuron" and the knowledge that it points to, physicians conceived "the nervous system to be composed of an aggregation of units very similar in character," and the challenge of neurology consisted of "the thorough study of these units." Brown continued, "It is important at the outset to have a name which shall appropriately designate this unit, and I have adopted Waldeyer's term of neuron to which, however Prof. Schäfer of London, objects; and while his reasons for putting forth a nomenclature of his own are sound, I think Waldeyer's term is so familiar and its application so readily understood and accepted that it will come into universal use."[14] And so it was. By 1899, the British neurologist William Gowers (1845–1915), who had first described the relevant lesions in "chronic progressive muscular atrophy" as affecting upper and lower "segments" of the motor path, was able to clarify his understanding of this pathology thanks to the neuron doctrine.

The upper segment, first diagrammed in Gower's *Manual of Nervous Diseases* (1886), links cortical cells (cells in the motor cortex) to the anterior gray column, via a pyramidal fiber; the diagram from 1886 shows a connected bundle linking the upper segment with the lower segment, beginning with a spinal cell, connected to muscle through a nerve fiber. The third (and last) edition of Gower's *Manual*, from 1899, included that same diagram but then showed Cajal's finding of the synaptic gap and by this point, on the threshold of the twentieth century, had incorporated the term "neuron." Gower's third edition was rewritten so as to restate how the cortex (in the brain) is linked to each muscle:

> Let us now consider, for a moment, the whole motor path, from the cortex of the brain to the muscles. *We may regard it as composed of two neurons, an upper and a lower.* Each consists of a ganglion-cell above, an axon, and the terminal ramification of the latter. The upper, "cerebrospinal," neuron consists of the cortical ganglion cell with its dendrons, and the "pyramidal axon" which proceeds from the cell, passes through the brain and cord, and ends in the grey substance by division and terminal interlacement with several nerve cells. The lower, "spinomuscular" neuron consists of the spinal motor cell with its dendrons and the axon proceeding from it, which passes through the anterior root and nerve-trunk to the muscle, where it divides and ramifies on

the muscular fibre. The elements of the two neurons do not correspond in number, since, as we have just seen, each cerebro-spinal element is connected with many spino-muscular elements. So too, each motor axon is connected with a considerable area of excitable muscle tissue. It will be found that this conception of the motor path conduces to clearer ideas of many facts of disease, and it is important to grasp it firmly.[15]

The change in anatomical understanding of the location of lesions and the affected cells certainly reinforced neurological knowledge of clinical signs to the degree that a language developed for understanding pathology in the living patient: spasticity and hyperreflexia not only were lateral column signs but, more specifically, became "upper motor neuron" signs; muscle wasting was then requalified as a sign of lower motor neuron degeneration.

But what about knowledge of the underlying disease?

The name "amyotrophic lateral sclerosis" was invented by Charcot in 1875 to distinguish it from other similar illnesses characterized by motor degeneration. As he said concerning Duchenne's term "glossolabial paralysis," it's a syndrome but not a diagnosis.

A diagnosis, in Charcot's eyes, required nosological clarity: the analytic act of separating forms of the disease was a way of knowing the illness. Others, principally Gowers, thought that such an *analytic* act in fact covered over knowing, or rather trying to know and understand (not the same thing) the *actual phenomenon* of the disease. For Gowers, Charcot's analytic work of disease categorization in fact obfuscated the question of its underlying biological cause, which is still unknown today.[16]

Over the 1840s and 1850s, clinicians concerned with cases of motor degeneration endeavored to analyze and categorize illnesses that resulted in both weakness and atrophy, a topic of increasing neurological interest. In 1850, the term *atrophie musculaire progressive* (progressive muscular atrophy) was used by François-Amilcar Aran (1817–1861) to describe patients with different patterns of progressive muscle weakness and atrophy of the limbs, patterns that Aran had collected from case reports recorded by Guillaume-Benjamin-Amand Duchenne (de Boulogne) (1806–1875).[17] Duchenne had described a case corresponding to what Aran would come to call progressive muscular atrophy, a year earlier, in 1849, and then carried on studying muscular atrophy and its connection to destruction of the cells in the anterior horn of the spinal cord "but was never sure which lesion occurred first."[18] In 1853, Jean Cruveilhier (1791–1874) "had noticed thinness of the anterior roots and spinal cord" in cases of atrophy, and "this was considered to be the essential lesion until Luys found degeneration of the anterior horn cells" in 1860.[19]

Put otherwise and reduced to its critical point, the search for the "essential" lesion still left open the question of causation: whether muscle wasting was caused by something happening in the muscle itself and then spreading out to the nerves or whether it was the other way around.

Only in 1891, thanks to the work of Wilhelm Heinrich Erb (1840–1921), would two distinct forms of atrophy be clearly distinguished, those that originate in the muscle tissue or the bone marrow. Charcot had understood that different kinds of nerve and muscular problems were included under the term "progressive muscular atrophy," and he endeavored and was able to distinguish different possible diagnoses within the same syndromic palate.

A theme can be raised from the sequence of discoveries that occurred between roughly 1811 and 1875, those discoveries by Bell, Aran-Duchenne, and Cruveilhier prior to Charcot's contribution to the specification of a distinct diagnosis for ALS: first, that one necessary condition for the emergence of a diagnosis was the formation of neurological concepts that could link both clinical and anatomopathological (empirical) knowledge. Without concepts and methods, terms such as "progressive muscular atrophy" or descriptions such as "weakness" would cover vastly different kinds of illness, and hence we would be in the terrain of syndromic description but not diagnosis.

For analysis and then diagnosis to take place, precise description of clinical signs had to be correlated to anatomical lesions. These topics have already been largely explored in the history of medicine, and so I return to them merely as preparation for my core concern, not only Charcot's concern regarding what use is a medicine that cannot provide amelioration, a question he raised at the end of his consultation in 1888, but moreover, *how to live with this knowledge at a time when no treatment is available*—a question for medical professionals, patients, and families alike, still today.

The question is all the more pertinent under conditions where Charcot's solution, to "let the patient live in illusion," is beyond the ethical pale today.

Sight and Site of Pathology

The coming into being of amyotrophic lateral sclerosis as an event in medical knowledge in the late nineteenth century is but a specific case of what Michel Foucault traced in his historical account of the emergence of the "medical gaze" in *The Birth of the Clinic*, namely, that it was only with the development of anatomopathological inquiry and methods that medicine "rediscovered analysis in the body itself."[20] Foucault already gave us a clear view of what changed over the early nineteenth century, and the change is exemplified in neurology: "Clinical experience sees a new space opening up before it: the tangible space of the body, which at the same time is that opaque mass in which secrets, invisible lesions, and the very mystery of origins lie hidden. The medicine of symptoms will gradually recede, until it finally disappears before the medicine of organs, sites, causes, before a clinic wholly ordered in accordance with pathological anatomy."[21] Foucault was excessive in his characterization of a sea change, to the degree that a medicine of symptoms did not disappear: indeed, he indicates as such with a qualification of his (overly) strong statement, reminding the reader that the clinician cannot be satisfied with the analysis of disease in death: "A clinic of symptoms seeks the living body of the disease; anatomy provides it only with the corpse."[22] In that clinic of symptoms, it is not only the medical gaze that seeks the living body of the disease, but first and foremost the one who is living with the body and the illness (an individual with a body, a person in a social form, a subject in and of speech) and who seeks to know what is happening to them.

The specificity of Charcot's work was precisely his search for and discovery of the sites, or rather, in the vocabulary of the time, the "seats" of pathology in the living body. As the neurologist and Charcot scholar Christopher G. Goetz points out, Charcot was, of course, not the first to use an anatomo-clinical method, but Charcot's unique contribution was through his application and development of it: "Because the method led to the discovery of a disease that had previously been unrecognized and it components confused, the history of Charcot's research efforts and application of his methodology is particularly revealing," Goetz wrote.[23]

Charcot's first discovery of anatomo-clinical significance to ALS was a case from 1865, a young woman, diagnosed as a hysteric, who developed weakness and increased muscle tone. Her intellect was preserved, there were no sensory issues, and urinary control was normal. Pathology showed the following:

> On careful examination of the surface of the spinal cord, on both sides in the lateral areas, there are two brownish grey streak marks produced by sclerotic changes. These grayish bands begin outside the line of insertion of the posterior roots and their anterior border approaches but does not include the entrance area of the anterior roots. They are visible throughout the thoracic region and continue, though greatly thinning out, up to the widening point of the cervical cord. Below, they are barely visible in the thoraco-lumbar region. Transverse sections taken at different levels allow one to see that the lateral columns have in their most superficial and posterior regions, a gray, semitransparent appearance, rather gelatinous. . . . At no point does the diseased tissue penetrate the gray matter which remains unaffected.[24]

Four years later, a paper published with his colleague Alix Joffroy (1844–1908) took up observations of cases of infantile paralysis without contractures, noting that only the anterior horns of the gray matter were affected.

Two observations, two correlations: lateral column lesions correlated to chronic progressive paralysis with contractures *and no muscle wasting*; anterior horn degeneration correlated to infantile paralysis *with muscle wasting*. Equipped with two observations, he tested the hypothesis that there was a two-part division of the motor system in the spinal cord between the lateral columns and the anterior columns. He confirmed Erb's observations of cases that were uniquely lateral (what would come to be called "primary lateral sclerosis") presenting with the same clinical features, as well as anterior horn cases, what would come to be known as cases of lower motor neuron only disease. Some cases, however, showed both.[25]

What is important to acknowledge is not only that Charcot established a direct relationship between a neurological lesion and a patient's clinical problem but also how he did so. In Goetz's terms, "a precise anatomic diagnosis could be given before death."[26] Charcot wrote, "In the beginning it was a matter of studying a series of cases primarily from an anatomic perspective. Nonetheless, the clinical characteristics of the patients had always been recorded carefully. Eventually among these different cases, it became possible to delineate a certain number of fundamental features, characteristics that permitted us later to recognize the condition clinically during life."[27] The tendency to hagiography when it comes to Charcot and the invention of the diagnostic category of amyotrophic lateral sclerosis has recently been allayed by reference to the British physician Jacob Augustus Lockhart Clarke's (1817–1880) contribution to the pathological description of the disease. Beyond the trivial issue of national rivalry, what is important about Clarke's contribution is that it underscores that Charcot was working in a broader field of neurological knowledge and a technical environment, especially histopathology, that rendered a specific kind of knowledge of motor diseases possible.

Clarke coauthored in 1862 "what appears to be an early detailed clinicopathological description of a case of ALS," published with Charles Bland Radcliffe (1822–1889) in the *British and Foreign Medico-Chirurgical Review*.[28] Radcliffe and Clarke concluded with respect to their histopathological inquiry:

> Looking at the clinical facts, it was obvious that there was no material injury in the seat of intelligence, and it was probable that there was some grave injury to the parts which rule the movements of the tongue and pharynx, and the respiratory movements generally. Without this latter injury, indeed, it was difficult to account for the palsied and wasted state

of the tongue, for the difficult deglutition, for the occasional trouble of breathing, for the mode of dying. All the most prominent symptoms of disease—the extensive paralysis and muscular atrophy described in the history of the patient, are so clearly and satisfactorily explained by the lesions of structure discovered on examination of the nervous centers, that the case now before us must be considered one of the most remarkable and interesting on record.[29]

They then suggested that "the ordinary and inefficient method of examining the nervous centers . . . would *perhaps have resulted in ranking the case as one of simple muscular atrophy.*"[30]

The detailed pathological examination of the nervous centers is a case in point of the first step toward how anatomopathological analysis could be connected to nosology.

As Foucault wrote regarding the birth of anatomopathological knowledge, "Two series of questions confront a pathological anatomy that wishes to be based on a nosology: the first concerns the connexion between a temporal set of symptoms and a spatial coexistence of tissues; the second concerns death and the strict definition of its relation to life and disease."[31] A response to this series of questions, Foucault explains, comes from the operation of comparison: the comparison of healthy anatomy with pathological anatomy, as well as the comparison of pathological cases of putatively similar illnesses. Clarke was able to provide the first response but not the second: "I was surprised to find that scarcely a vestige could be seen of the large groups of cells which are found in corresponding parts of the healthy cord . . . the cells were wonderfully altered from their natural appearance . . . looked like aggregated granules . . . all more or less atrophied and shriveled."[32] Clarke went on to describe the anterior horn cell and corticospinal tract degeneration that would come to be known as characteristic of ALS: "All the white columns of the cord in every region, but particularly in the cervical region, had suffered more or less from atrophy or degeneration . . . the anterior roots of the nerves were decidedly below their average size."[33] He then moved to the brainstem: "From about the lower end of the olivary bodies to the commencement of the fourth ventricle, the morbid changes were much greater and more extensive. . . . The hypoglossal or lingual nerve-roots in their course through the medulla, were also in places not more than half their natural size; and in other places could scarcely be discerned."[34] Observations of a single case gave a firm pathological indication for the continued search for a diagnostic category, to be provided later by Charcot.

With respect to this exemplary achievement of anatomo-clinical medicine, what is modified, according to Foucault, "is not, therefore, the mere surface of contact between the knowing subject and the known object; it is the more general arrangement of knowledge that determines the reciprocal positions and the connexion *between the one who must know and that which is to be known*."[35] Let us recall, nevertheless, that the cause(s) of the syndrome are still to this day unknown: a medicine of organs and sites has been ever increasingly specified without a corresponding traction on the problem of cause, thus returning medical care and patient experience to the surface of their everyday symptoms.

What is crucial to recall, therefore, is that there is a movement between site, of disease and death, and surface signs, of the living body, for the individual: a traction or movement back and forth that endeavors to know the truth of the disease and, more important, to ask how to *live* with knowledge of illness when there is little prospect of ameliorating the progression of the disease itself.

That which is to be known, in other words, is a dual object of attention, *the truth of the disease* that could one day lead to cure, and *the truth of the illness*, which can only be approached as the practical question of how to live with it, when there is nothing to stop it.

Between 1840 and 1899, that which was to be known was the anatomic correlation between localizable lesions and clinical signs. "The one who must know," to use Foucault's phrase, was oriented, as with Lockhart Clark and Charcot, to the side and site of death, to see the sites of death in the living. Knowing, for Charcot, meant analyzing signs and linking them to locatable anatomical lesions, linkages that would then distinguish disease types depending on whether there was only muscle wasting, only spasticity and hyperreflexia, or both. This knowledge is remarkably stable constituting the core of a diagnosis today.

Of crucial importance, however, in the history of knowledge of this illness is that on the one hand, this analytic orientation, this deductive reasoning, provides a clarity of procedure for diagnosis that continues to this day, and yet, the lack of knowledge about etiology returns everyone concerned, and foremost the patient themselves, to the constellation of symptoms, which become part of a life.

Such a return to the heterogeneous character of the syndrome is reflected in the way that ALS today is a word with multiple referents: extremity onset, bulbar onset, lower motor neuron only, and whether someone with primary lateral sclerosis (PLS, upper motor neuron only symptoms) will "convert" at some point (frequently the case), thus rendering for some neurologists the very category of PLS questionable. What matters, though, is not the category per se but (one might think) rather care for the patient's symptoms, and what matters in terms of knowledge is trying to understand the biological cause.

Gowers, in his 1899 overview of "chronic spinal muscular atrophy," a term he preferred to Charcot's term, underscores that frequently what appears as lower motor neuron only disease often, "in a very large proportion of cases," involves pyramidal tract degeneration (upper motor neuron degeneration), such that "Charcot's distinction is in effect giving a new name to an old disease."[36] Underscoring the variability and heterogeneity of clinical manifestation, he wrote, "Whether there are indications of lateral sclerosis or not, depends on the circumstance whether the degeneration of the pyramidal fibers is or is not more extensive than the complete degeneration of the nerve cells that causes atonic atrophy."[37] Further on, he wrote,

> The pyramidal tracts may be totally degenerated, and yet there may be none of the characteristic indications of such degeneration. On the other hand, both arms and legs may be the seat of the spastic paralysis that indicates pyramidal degeneration, and atonic atrophy may be limited to a few muscles of the hands. Between these we have every gradation of degree and distribution of atonic atrophy, spastic paralysis, and tonic wasting. Of these only the last named indicates an affection of the gray matter secondary, in point of time, to the pyramidal degeneration, and even then only in part secondary in point of causation. *Hence a division into two classes (into which the same case may fall at different periods) is less in harmony with the facts of disease, than is a recognition of the varying extent of the lesion and the corresponding variation of clinical character and course.*[38]

What mattered to Gowers was not whether he could make distinctions between classes of symptoms. Rather, what mattered to him was to grasp the clinical phenomena so as to be able to inquire into the underlying biology that went into producing those phenomena, cognizant of the fact that the same phenotype may be caused by multiple different biological operations: it was also known to Gowers that at autopsy in ALS, there are always many preserved anterior horn cells; indeed, "the process of motor neuronal loss is strikingly patchy and multifocal, despite the more demarcated and sequential spread of symptoms reported by patients."[39]

In the United Kingdom, following Gowers, the syndromic understanding of the disease was reflected in a new name, "motor neuron disease," used by Russell Brain in his textbook *Clinical Neurology* and his *Diseases of the Nervous System* from roughly the 1960s. Summarizing Gowers's view, Brain wrote in 1962 that there are two varieties of progressive muscular atrophy, one characterized only by lower motor neuron lesions and one with symptoms of corticospinal tract lesions: "These two varieties are now usually regarded as nosologically similar. Greenfield [1958] preferred the term amyotrophic lateral sclerosis to motor neurone disease on the grounds that the pathological changes in the spinal cord are not limited to the motor neurons and many American authors use this term as an inclusive one, embracing all varieties of the disease. Motor neurone disease, however, is a better inclusive term."[40] Regardless, the curiosity, if not tension, is that while all agree on motor neuron disease/ALS as constituting a syndrome, within the heterogeneous assemblage of signs, the question of whether distinct diseases can be distinguished, or not, does not seem to go away. It does not go away for a very simple reason: there is, at least in part, a desire to know and a desire that knowledge could be connected to how a person lives with illness: lower or upper only diseases tend to progress more slowly, and bulbar presentations are quickly highly debilitating. The patient, at least at the moment of looking for a diagnosis, wishes to know something about why they are not well.

While this chapter has endeavored to show the emergence of a relatively stable diagnostic category, this story will be intersected with a parallel narrative to be opened up in the chapter that follows. I trace a second step in the history of this illness as the syndromic understanding of disease expands to include cognitive or "mental" aspects, thus posing the question of the degree to which motor neuron disease is *only* a motor neuron disease and confusing the relation between clinical phenotypical presentation and the underlying biological mechanisms.

NOSOLOGICAL INDETERMINATIONS

Pierre Marie (1853–1940), the French neurologist who would come to occupy Charcot's position at the Hôpital Salpêtrière, noted something original about ALS in his *Lectures on Diseases of the Spinal Cord*, published in 1892—namely, a "mental" or cognitive aspect to the illness, what he termed a "decrease of mental power":

> Before ending these remarks upon the nature of amyotrophic lateral sclerosis allow me, gentlemen, to insist once more upon the fact that more than one point of contact seems to exist between this disease and the forms of general paresis of the insane, to which I have just alluded, and in which degeneration of the pyramidal tracts, which is limited to the cord, is observed to occur. Analogies exist as regards the pathological anatomy; *the clinical condition shows indisputable decrease of mental power in every case of amyotrophic lateral sclerosis, even when the indication of paresis and atrophy seem confined to the limbs*; these seem to me good reasons for comparing these two morbid conditions with each other. It must be well understood, gentlemen, that *I do not consider these two diseases as identical or even analogous from a clinical point of view*, but am convinced that they should be placed close to each other if merely considered in connection with general topographical nosography.[1]

Such mental or cognitive symptoms had not been mentioned by Charcot as characteristic of, or coincident with, the illness. Both prior authors and, it must be emphasized, later authors have been explicit about this disease being specific to motor degeneration, and hence they explicitly considered the disease as attacking neither the sensory pathway nor cognition-related parts of the nervous system.

From the turn of the twentieth century, however, the interlinking of motor neuron disease/ALS and cognitive issues would continue to intensify, and toward the century's end, in 1990, British neurologist David Neary and his colleagues in Manchester came to (under)state that the "nosological status" of the co-occurrence of different kinds of dementias with motor neuron disease was increasingly taken up as an object of inquiry and yet considered still riddled with indetermination.[2]

Beginning with Pierre Marie in 1892, however, the cognitive issues observed in tandem with ALS were diffuse, and Marie would not let his clinical observations of disease, his nosography, disrupt or question ALS nosology, its classification. He stated, in a footnote that accompanied the above citation, that he could not admit "as some authors have maintained, that amyotrophic lateral sclerosis, progressive muscular atrophy, and the different forms of myopathy are varieties of one process alone, *rings, as it were, of the same chain*. Important differences exist between them while very few analogies bring them together."[3] What is curious is how these two points are connected: on the one hand, Marie was making a clinical observation about the range of symptoms that can appear in patients diagnosed with ALS, symptoms that include cognitive issues, which had not previously been discussed in the neurological literature. On the other hand, because of the connection he noted between general "paresis of the insane"—dementia paralytica—and ALS, their contiguous placement in a "general topographical nosography," which is to say their proximate location on a map, or plane, of disease descriptions, he was therefore compelled to make the point that although he recognized the close relation of ALS to other diseases, diseases that Charcot had been at pains to distinguish from ALS, he did not therefore consider various kinds of paralysis and muscular weakness to be part of "one process alone," as he put it.

I underscore the point, as well as the connection between these two thoughts, because they are at the heart of an indetermination in knowledge about ALS, one that grew in intensity over twelve decades and remains with us today. The indetermination turns on the question of whether there is a single pathological process underlying ALS, a process that could moreover explain the links between ALS and cognitive issues. Hence, the indetermination is a subtle one: although it looks to be only about whether "ALS patients are cognitively normal," in fact this starting point also then opens out onto a bigger indetermination of what, biologically speaking, is/are this/these disease(s).

Such a concern is precisely what has come to be at stake in the history of the expansion of what may or may not be said to be a co-occurrence (a *syn-drome*) and is at stake in the endeavor to explain the biological mechanisms underlying ALS, which are supposed to account for both neuromuscular degeneration and cognitive decline.

Concretely: Are psychoses, dementias, language function issues, and mood disorders part of ALS as a disease, or do they instead simply index comorbid disease processes and coincident symptoms? Is there one biological process that manifests in several ways?

My concern here is not, of course, to arbitrate by way of biomedical judgment but rather to track how, at different moments over the changing history of knowledge of ALS, this question has been posed and how inquirers have endeavored to answer it, as well as the open question of the significance of any response to such inquiries for knowledge of the illness. What I will not provide is a full account of the state of molecular biological knowledge about ALS in the present, not only because of my own limitations in terms of molecular biological competence but also, and more important, because of the still highly disjointed molecular biological knowledge of the illness.

Broadly speaking, the history of the expansion of ALS as a syndrome to include mental or cognitive issues, within medical knowledge, can be tracked schematically through four historical moments, each one raising questions as to how to take up and link together the heterogeneity of signs, particularly cognitive signs, with ideas about what kind of neurodegeneration is involved: an association, a complex, an overlap, and an integration—these are the four different ways of taking up and interlinking the assemblage of neurodegeneration and cognitive issues. Each moment at which ALS and cognitive issues are considered together reconfigures the assemblage of signs whose "topographical nosography" indicates their placement on a single surface but lacks an overarching and consistent conceptualization.

Overview of Four Moments of Interconnection between ALS and Cognitive Issues

In order to assist the reader in following what is a highly complex series of historical moments, or phases, I first provide an overview of each moment, underscoring both the historical timing and the manner in which the motor illness is considered related to neuropsychiatric or cognitive issues.

1892–1932: Association of Signs

An association of signs and a coincidence of diseases from psychosis to Pick's disease: The initial association of pure motor signs with signs of cognitive and behavioral degeneration in the 1890s is later specified, from around 1930, with reference to particular psychiatric and neurodegenerative illnesses. The majority of authors during this first moment consider psychosis to be coincidental, although other cognitive or affect issues, such as mood problems or emotional lability, were (and are still today) considered mental troubles caused by the neurodegenerative illness itself. Today, such emotional lability is called "pseudobulbar affect"—excessive/easy laughter/crying, for which there is now a medication Nudexta, approved by the Food and Drug Administration (FDA) in 2010. A specific neurodegenerative illness, Pick's disease, was noted for the first time in 1932 as presenting along with ALS. The illness is named after Czech neuropsychiatrist Arnold Pick, who in 1892 began to publish a series of cases through which he argued for the cognitive, semantic, and behavioral effects of focal atrophy and lesions in the temporal and frontal lobes. The term "Pick atrophy" was introduced in 1922 by A. Gans to refer to the connection between frontal lobe atrophy and a description of a kind of senile dementia that could not be explained in vascular terms and that had a hereditary disposition. The term "Pick's disease" was used by K. Onari and H. Spatz in 1926, later to be reclassified in the 1990s under a more general banner of "frontotemporal dementias." As with psychosis, the association of Pick's disease with ALS was at that time considered an association of two independent illnesses. This hypothesis of coincidence would come to be questioned as a more integrated view of the clinical tableau was developed with reference to underlying biology.

1945–1990: Disease Complex

A disease complex—ALS and parkinsonism-dementia on the island of Guam: Beginning in 1945, a chance and surprising observation by American physicians of an endemic focus of both ALS and parkinsonism-dementia on the island of Guam, with a high percentage of patients presenting with a mixture of symptoms of both illnesses, with traceable family histories, led to the exploration of a series of genetic and environmental hypotheses about the causes of these illnesses and the underlying biological mechanisms. The very high rates of disease noted during this period eventually trailed off from the 1980s onward, indicating a likely environmental cause. The case ultimately produced more questions than answers, marking a further layer of indetermination in which a link between heterogeneous dementias and ALS was both clearly marked out and little understood. The anatomopathological inquiries at autopsy led to a confidence, in the 1960s, among some neurologists as to the hypothesis of an underlying biological process uniting the two illnesses, parkinsonism-dementia and ALS, especially given the initial genetic hypothesis. Indetermination, however, remained high, given the lack of biological knowledge.[4]

1980–2011: Anatomo-Molecular Overlap

Anatomo-clinical, histopathological, and molecular overlap between (Pick's) fron-totemporal lobar degeneration and ALS and the claim to a spectrum disorder: Anatomopathological and imaging studies in ALS populations confirmed the involvement of cerebral pathology beyond the motor cortex, including in the temporal and frontal lobes, and clinical studies began to increasingly pay attention to, and hence observe, subtle dysexecutive symptoms and increasing reports of patients presenting with both ALS and the renamed "frontotemporal dementias" (renamed in the 1990s). Despite building on the work of small groups of researchers who, over the 1950s, 1960s, and 1970s, tracked not only Pick's disease, a dementia that came to be slowly distinguished from Alzheimer's-type dementia, but also the co-occurrence of ALS and Pick's, the nosological status of dementias with ALS remained unclear. With respect to this indetermination, what can be traced are the strategies through which clarification of the problem of classification was attempted and how clinical observation of the overlap increasingly supported a view that ALS and frontotemporal dementias are a spectrum of a single disorder. The 2006 publication of a shared neuropathological signature of cytoplasmic ubiquitinated inclusions of the protein TDP-43 in ALS and frontotemporal dementia (FTD) gave a molecular reason for the link observed between the two illnesses. A second molecular finding from 2011 showed a "strong association" of a hexonucleotide repeat expansion on chromosome 9 with autosomal dominant inherited FTD and ALS. By 2018, Raul Desikan, a neuroradiologist who had been researching the overlap between multiple kinds of neurodegenerative illness and was diagnosed in 2017 with ALS, published, with his colleague Celeste Karch, a meta-genome-wide association study that showed ALS shares risk factors with diseases of the FTD spectrum, including supranuclear palsy and corticobasal degeneration, and that no shared variants were found in ALS and Parkinson's or ALS and Alzheimer's disease.

1900/2000: Integration

An integrating hypothesis of neurodegeneration: Finally, there has recently been an effort to provide an "integrative" narrative that incorporates the history of the links between dementias and ALS into an operable model of functional connections between motor and cognitive degeneration, in order to account for the selective degeneration along those functional paths. Such an integrative account draws on both the old and the new, seeking a contemporary understanding of ALS that aims at providing a coherent explanation and yet remains speculative.

A Nosological Question

Whereas during the nineteenth century, anatomopathology was the decisive tool for knowing ALS, today, the molecular biological underpinnings of the various clinical signs, along with neuroimaging and neuropathological findings, are the means through which hypotheses are made about the possibility that a variety of neurodegenerative illnesses stem from common underlying disease processes. The indetermination and challenge is then to integrate the clinical, pathological, and molecular understandings of ALS.

The indetermination is curious and worth exploring to the degree that support for an expanded clinical understanding of ALS to include cognitive issues has not yet resulted in a change to classification or diagnostic procedure. To put it squarely: cognitive issues are not determinant in making a diagnosis of ALS, and motor issues are not taken into account when making a diagnosis of behavioral-variant frontotemporal dementia.[5] Nevertheless, the more than century-long discussion of the overlap has, as Pierre Marie noted already in 1892, given reason to locate these illnesses contiguously on a plane and hence to then pose the question of the underlying mechanisms that explain their proximity, as well as to prepare caregivers for the tribulations of such a symptomatic doubling.

This question, moreover, is being approached, today, through molecular biological knowledge of genetic overlap between these illnesses and a biological understanding of the multiple disease mechanisms involved, some of which are shared by multiple illnesses.

Otherwise said, there is still a disjunction between knowledge of illness as it presents in the clinic and knowledge of molecular disruption that is thought to cause the illness. The gap between clinical and biological knowledge is not of the same kind as the gap between, say, anatomo-clinical knowledge of glioblastoma and the biological causes of such brain tumors, to give one point of comparison.

The difference lies in the degree to which knowledge of underlying biological cause, in the case of ALS and cognitive-affective-behavioral issues, has the capacity to reconfigure the very nature of what the disease is thought to be. It is relative to these two sites and forms of knowledge, a clinical form and molecular biological form that an "integrative" narrative endeavors to give coherence today.

1892–1932: An Association of Signs and Coincidence of Diseases: From Psychosis to Pick's Disease

One of Pierre Marie's students, Marius Bordes, wrote his medical thesis on *Considérations sur les troubles psychiques dans le tabes, dans la sclérose en plaques et dans la sclérose latérale amyotrophique* [*Reflections on Psychic Disorders in Tabes (Dorsalis), Multiple Sclerosis and Amyotrophic Lateral Sclerosis*].[6] A synthetic work from 1908, it drew on Marie's brief observations, as well as on the clinical work of Alexandre Cullerre (1849–1934), the then director of the asylum at La Roche-sur-Yon. Concerning Marie's observations of a link between "mental troubles" and ALS, Bordes quotes Marie stating that he considered such troubles not only as frequent but moreover as "constituting one of the usual symptoms." Strictly speaking, Marie wrote, the alterations of psychic functions are not obvious,

> but if we take the trouble to look for them, we will find, almost certainly, a propensity to laugh or cry without just cause; emotionality will be extremely exaggerated; besides, the intellectual and moral disposition [*l'habitus*] of the patient will have assumed a childlike aspect; his credulity, his silliness will sometimes be quite singular.[7]

Bordes continued, summarizing his observations from a clinical case:

> To these dementia and affective disorders are added transient melancholic raptures, with fits of despair and sudden impulses to suicide, which have occurred more or less frequently throughout the course of the disease. . . . Then, the patient is sequestrated, his emotional perversions find new nourishment in his tense relations with the nurses responsible for caring for him; then flourishes a veritable delusion of persecution that we would be tempted to describe as senile, but for his age, so much delirium resembles that which is commonly observed in old men with cortical lesions. . . . As in all organic psychopathies, a

separation must be made in the psychopathological manifestations observed in this patient: on the one hand, the dementia symptoms, deficit disorders, due to the early involvement in the cortex of lesions that fall under amyotrophic lateral sclerosis; on the other hand, psychic symptoms which are only the manifestation of a particular predisposition of the subject.[8]

Importantly, the emergence of a cognitive aspect to the illness allows for attention to the individual, an individual with their physiology that manifests the illness, a self with their particular psychic predispositions, a person with their relations and biography, their personal history, and not only a body that succumbs to the mechanics of motor degeneration.

In the first case that Bordes reproduces, a case of mental disorder connected with ALS, taken from Cullerre's clinical observations, the exam history and the classification of the patient on entry into the asylum indicate "delirium consequent to chronic myelitis"—which is inflammation of the spinal cord. Gowers had cautioned prudence when he stated in his *Manual* (1899) that "there has been a tendency in recent pathology to extend the conception of inflammation so as to include all morbid processes which do not consist in an actual new growth. The extension is chiefly based on the difficulty of drawing a dividing line between inflammation and other processes."[9] In the case of this patient, Pierre, a forty-seven-year-old railway worker who entered the asylum at the end of summer 1903, such a caution had been heeded, and after twenty-one hours, the delirium consequent to chronic myelitis had been requalified as "organic dementia (amyotrophic lateral sclerosis) with hallucinations, persecution delirium and agitated impulsive outbursts."[10] His family history indicated that his father died of epilepsy and his mother of an unknown illness. Pierre contracted gonorrhea at age thirty-five, complicated by rheumatoid arthritis and double iritis: syphilis was ruled out. A few years later, another episode of gonorrhea and again iritis with adhesions, which altered his vision. He was forced to undergo a double iridectomy, despite which he could not go back to work. Moreover, he had a number of problems with the authorities concerning his pension, and it is relative to these difficulties that Pierre's sister attributed the onset of the illness for which he was confined and which progressed over a period of three years. The case report continues:

> Lower extremity paralysis; tongue paralysis; to a lesser degree the arms; severe changes in mood. He took a dislike to his sister who cared for him, imagining that she wanted to get rid of him and take his possessions. He showers her with insults, has outbursts of childish excitement

with uncontrollable spasmodic crying, hallucinations and tried several times to commit suicide by throwing himself out the window or down the well of the house. As soon as he entered the asylum, he showed a constant emotionality, puerile demands and great irritability. He complains about everyone, he refuses the food provided, only willing to take what comes from home; he accuses the nurses of brutality, insults them and threatens revenge. He wishes to be armed with his cane at all times, to be able to defend himself against his sister whom he constantly sees before him, claiming that she wants to seize his money to maintain a lover. He insults her with horrible names: ". . . penniless whore, you are very happy to have found me so as to live at my expense," etc. When she comes to see him, on the contrary, he shows an overt satisfaction, caresses and expressions of friendship; then, as soon as she has turned her back, he begins again his litany of insults, especially when he has exhausted the provision of snacks, which she does not fail to bring him . . . October 1903. Rampage of persecution more intense than ever . . . March 1904. The attacks of asphyxia become more and more frequent, he cannot eat without the greatest difficulties, gnawing at every bite. He succumbs April 11 to the progress of asphyxiation.[11]

Bordes reproduces several other case histories of mental troubles with paralysis and makes the following, very general, conclusion:

Just as cerebral affections—such as general paralysis, for example—cause spinal cord lesions, so spinal disorders frequently cause brain damage [cerebral lesions]. It is not surprising, then, that the diseases of the cord are almost always accompanied by mental disorders. If the pyramidal cell is affected, we can have all the signs of cerebral insufficiency, from slight decrease in psychic activity to dementia. If the medullary disease affects both the cerebral cortex and the meninges, paralytic syndrome is observed. Finally, when the bulbar nuclei and the conductive bundles of psycho-mimetic innervation in the oval center, the internal capsule and the bulb are injured, there may be spasmodic laughter and crying, without concordance of intellectual disturbances.[12]

It must be underscored nevertheless that what "accompaniment" means in the above citation—"diseases of the cord are almost always accompanied by mental disorders"—remains an open question. Moreover, it is of concern as to how to characterize what is specific to the disorder and what is specific to the person, their disposition, or predisposition: "The deliriums of this medullary affection resemble the psychoses of old age. As in other organic psychopathies, one must see in the dementia complications of amyotrophic lateral sclerosis a consequence of the organic lesion and, in delirious manifestations, a consequence of the [individual's] predisposition."[13] Bordes's general orientation is later specified with more effort at anatomopathological correlation, to discern further the symptoms that are consequent to organic lesion and those consequent to individual pre-disposition or some other process. The Belgian neurologist Ludo van Bogaert (1897–1989) "thought that psychosis with amyotrophic lateral sclerosis might be due to cerebral lesions. However, . . . [van Bogaert] did not believe that a diag-nosis of amyotrophic lateral sclerosis could be made on the basis of the psychic disturbances which were, nevertheless, worthy of much interest."[14] Broadly speaking during this first moment 1892–1932, we can see that five classes of "mental" symptoms were raised by neurologists in their connection with the stan-dard tableau of ALS: (1) deliria/psychosis, (2) easy laughter/crying, (3) language pathology distinct from the motor issue of forming the actual words, (4) affect issues (depression; suicidal ideation), and (5) behavioral issues (incongruous/strange behaviors). For each class of symptom, the question becomes whether there is reason to link the symptom to ALS as a disease entity.

Regarding psychosis, the meaning of the term and the loose association was not further specified, and neurologists wavered between considering such delir-ium as coincidental with, or else as due to, a lesion produced by the disease. By contrast, "explosive emotional reactions," "emotional lability," and what came to be known later in neurological language as pseudobulbar affect—uncontrollable inappropriate laughter or crying—were already considered neurological issues due to lesions of the upper motor neurons that end in the nuclei.[15] Easy laughter and crying, which were already noted by Marie and initially considered a "mental" issue, were later qualified as "organic emotionalism." Pseudobulbar af-fect is the clearest instance of a "mental" sign being *strictly caused* by specific neurological degeneration that is part of the disease process of ALS. Moreover, the status of a patient's emotions needed to be approached with caution, to gather how, if at all, explosive emotional *reactions* were considered to be accompanied by the experience of the actual emotions. As Ziegler wrote in 1930,

> Wilson critically reviewed previous theories regarding pathologic laughing and weeping, but summarized them by saying that the tracts controlling these voluntary or involuntary movements are not known but are probably separate. This raises questions concerning the neuro-anatomic basis of emotions and their control which are far from set-tled. The subject deserves much study. Most textbooks on neuro-anatomy and neurophysiology concede that those upper motor neurons that end

in the nuclei of the brain stem have their origin in the Betz cells of the motor cortex. Herrick cited evidence that neurons from widely distributed areas of the cerebral cortex make synaptic connections with the nuclei in the brain stem. It seems clear, in some cases, that the emotions themselves are not changed, but that the motor reactions resembling those seen in well-defined emotional reactions behave as an ankle clonus or an overactive, easily elicited reflex.[16]

Hence an emotional problem was considered in motor terms as being consequent to the illness. With respect to affect issues and depression, Ziegler notes that a tendency to episodes of depression and euphoria has been noted in the literature. "Later in the course of the disease," he continued, "speechlessness and impoverishment of the usual intellectual processes (sometimes called dementia) were apparent. Disorientation did not seem uncommon."[17]

A pair of cases shows the ways in which behavioral issues (a case from Ziegler 1930) and language involvement (a case from Wechsler and Davison (1931) were considered, already in the early part of the twentieth century, as being included within the syndrome of ALS:

> A woman, aged 59, came to the Mayo Clinic in August, 1926, because of weakness in the legs of nine months' duration. Her mother had died of a "stroke" at the age of 50. The patient probably had had acute appendicitis at the age of 25. The menopause had come at the age of 50. About nine months before she came to the clinic she had noticed weakness and stiffness in the right leg, associated with some aching pain in the lumbosacral region, which extended up the spinal column. The weakness extended to the other leg and to the left arm. Four months previously, she had had some teeth extracted and had experienced annoying tremulousness and twitching under the skin throughout the body. She lost about 20 pounds (9 kg) in weight thereafter and became irritable, fearing that she would become paralyzed, a condition she had always dreaded. . . . The sensory examination gave negative results. The gait was spastic. The extremities were moderately weak. Examination of the spinal fluid gave negative results. The patient was often angry at a sister who came with her, and she wept spasmodically while angry. She could not be tolerant of her disability and fretted continually about it. She was oriented. A diagnosis of psychoneurotic reactions associated with amyotrophic lateral sclerosis was made. Within the next six months, the patient's physician reported that she grew worse and became spastic, and that signs of bulbar lesions became

pronounced. She had marked insomnia, was irritable, used vile, obscene and profane language, shrieked day and night, struck and tried to bite those who came near her and spat at friends and relatives and into her food. Her attending physician and the relatives declared that she was the hardest patient to care for they had ever seen. It was thought that she was oriented for place and person. It became necessary to place her in a state hospital; there her neurologic disabilities grew so profound as to preclude a diagnosis of psychosis. She died on Aug. 15, 1929. Necropsy was not obtained.[18]

In commenting on the cases, Ziegler notes, in keeping with the outlook that we have seen from Bordes and others, that "individual susceptibility to such reactions would vary greatly, so that early in the disease they would be manifested by certain patients, whereas by others they would not be shown even late in the ravages of the disease. That the disease may progress from toxic delirium to irreparable dementia due to intracranial lesions, seems apparent from its nature. It is further presumed that the psychosis and spasmodic emotional reactions probably bear a significant relation to the previous personality of the patients, and that these have been inadequately studied."[19] Wechsler and Davison reported on a Mr. H. L., noting something relatively underreported in case histories, namely, specific language issues:[20]

Mr. H. L., a man, aged 38, married, a fruit peddler, who was admitted to the Montefiore Hospital on Jan. 2, 1930, in November 1927, had begun to show mental changes characterized essentially by impairment of memory. The family noticed that he was "tongue-tied," reiterated statements without being aware of what he said, could not recall the names of his parents and failed to recognize the members of his family or the house and street in which he lived. He was unkempt, unconcerned, somewhat hesitant and stammering. In June, 1928, the patient was seen by a neurologist, who found atrophy of the arms and hands. At Mount Sinai Hospital, where he was from Oct. 5 to 28, 1928, a diagnosis of amyotrophic lateral sclerosis was made. He gradually became worse: his face became expressionless, he grew more careless about his person, at times he went without clothes, and he urinated any place about the house.—The patient was neglectful of his personal appearance. He knew his name, and repeated it three or four times at irregular intervals when asked for it. He was congenial but not capable of cooperating. He appeared slightly interested in his surroundings as long as there were variations, but this interest soon waned. He would answer questions occasionally with either "yes" or his name. He was disoriented for place and person. He wandered aimlessly about the ward, smiled fatuously and reacted to no particular situations.

Owing to his inaccessibility, an accurate study of the mental content and intellectual capacity could not be made. The inability to express himself was more than a dysarthria and partook of some degree of aphasia in addition to a profound intellectual deterioration. His affective responses were inappropriate. The mental picture resembled in the main an advanced dementia.

Autopsy and microscopic analysis were available, leading to the following commentary: "Clinically, in the case of [H. L.] there were two syndromes: (1) nuclear involvement, mainly of the bulb and upper part of the spinal cord, and pyramidal tract disease; these constitute the syndrome of amyotrophic lateral sclerosis; (2) a cerebral degenerative process characterized by mental deterioration (childishness, stubbornness, lack of cooperation, emotional instability and a tendency to euphoria and aphasia). The mental picture somewhat resembled Alzheimer's disease, though there was little to substantiate this, and certainly the anterior horn cell syndrome is foreign to it." The authors conclude, "In the vast majority of recorded cases, amyotrophic lateral sclerosis is not characterized clinically by definite psychotic manifestations. Most of the cases with such manifestations reported in the literature can better be explained by an incidental association with schizophrenic, manic-depressive or paranoid syndromes or with simple depressions. In older patients the occurrence of definite organic dementia could with more reason be ascribed to the coexistent, but at the same time independent, general cerebral arteriosclerosis."[21]

Such was also the case with Pick's disease. In 1932, for the first time, a German neurologist Von Braunmuhl described a clinical case of Pick's disease connected with motor neuron degeneration, the illness initially presenting with delusions of grandeur. Pick's disease is a syndrome of nonspecific frontal lobe degeneration, "known also as the frontal variant of fronto-temporal degeneration and presenting with marked changes in personality and behavior."[22] In this case, the ALS was considered by Von Braunmuhl as being secondary to Pick's and late in arrival. Anatomically, he reported an intense frontal atrophy, a minimal atrophy of the motor cortex, pyramidal damage, and damage to the anterior cornua of the marrow. Von Braunmuhl considered them two distinct processes, a confluence (however unlikely) of two rare illnesses.[23]

1945–1990: A Disease Complex: ALS and Parkinsonism-Dementia on the Island of Guam

The observation that ALS could present in a complex with dementias, whether Pick's, as in the reported case from 1932, or something that "somewhat resembled Alzheimer's disease," as in the case of H. L., was reinforced in 1961 with the publication of a paper "Parkinsonism-Dementia Complex, An Endemic Disease on the Island of Guam," in the influential journal *Brain*. The research, undertaken by Asao Hirano, Leonard Kurland, and others, was consequent to a chance and surprising discovery from 1945. As World War II wound down, Yale pathologist Harry M. Zimmerman (1901–1994) arrived on the southernmost Mariana Island as part of a Navy medical unit; "five months later, he sent an urgent report to his commanding officer, saying he had seen seven or eight civilians hospitalized with amyotrophic lateral sclerosis. The fatal illness seemed to be shockingly common."[24] All cases seemed to affect the indigenous Chamorro population but not other groups on the island. In 1949, Arthur Arnold, Donald Edgren, and Vincent Palladino, who were also on active duty with the US Navy between October 1947 and March 1949, published a short article documenting "ALS: Fifty Cases Observed on Guam." The incidence of 1:510 contrasted shockingly with the then US incidence rate approximated as 1:50,000. Familial occurrence was noted in five cases; "no obvious toxic agents were noted."[25]

Importantly, at this stage, the scientific and medical urgency stemmed from ALS focus and the possibility that the Guam case study could provide insights into a genetic variant of ALS. No mention was made in the paper of coincident parkinsonism-dementia. Kurland and his colleague D. W. Mulder would go on to investigate familial aggregations in a 1955 paper leading to a suggestion of "genetic influence," noteworthy in part because the genetic hypothesis would come to fall out of, and then back into, consideration: "Although familial aggregation of cases might be due to a common environmental factor as well as to a genetic influence, the distribution of cases among the various peoples in the area is more suggestive of a genetic influence than of an environmental factor. . . . Since the Guam findings suggested a hereditary rather than an external causative factor, we decided to reevaluate thoroughly the possible genetic factors in classical amyotrophic lateral sclerosis."[26] The authors reviewed the literature, making the point that at that time, the consensus was that familial forms are exceptionally rare.

A year earlier, in 1954, Mulder, Kurland, and local medic L. L. Iriarte conducted a house-to-house survey, focusing on ALS, but were attentive to the presentation of all forms of neurodegenerative illness.[27] Under the heading "Differential Diagnosis," they wrote, "In the course of this survey we examined many patients with neurologic disease other than amyotrophic lateral sclerosis. Often these patients came to our attention because the nurse or relative was unable to differentiate their condition from ALS. During the course of our study, 22 patients with parkinsonism were examined. In most instances the parkinsonism was believed to be postencephalitic in origin and the syndrome seemed similar to that which one of us (D.W.M) had described as following an epidemic of western equine encephalitis."[28] As work continued on Guam, the postencephalitic hypothesis was reconsidered. Asao Hirano, who worked under the supervision of Zimmerman, arrived on Guam in 1959. He and his colleagues began to systematically note cases in which signs of ALS were coincident with signs of parkinsonism-dementia.

> According to the reports at the Neurological Research Center on Guam, 21 additional cases with Parkinsonism, most of whom also had dementia, were observed during 1957 and 1958. A case register was established in late 1958 to facilitate a longterm prospective genetic investigation of ALS and Parkinsonism, and with the arrival of one of us (A. Hirano) on Guam in 1959, a concerted effort was made to provide a detailed clinical and pathological description of the cases. It soon became apparent that although a few patients had clinical features of Parkinson's disease, the large majority had a combination of a severe progressive dementia with extrapyramidal disease (Parkinsonism-dementia complex) and, in an appreciable number of patients, motor neurone involvement as well.[29]

In terms of the local knowledge of the presentation and coincidence of the illnesses, they were known to the Chamorro people as *Lytico-Bodig*: *lytico* (stemming from the Spanish *paralytico*) refers to those who have progressive paralysis and *bodig* (the Chamorro word for listless) to those whose condition resembled parkinsonism, often with dementia.

Hirano and colleagues noted, in their 1961 paper,

> striking akinesia and mask-like, expressionless face with a 'reptilian stare.' Coordination, alternating movement, and skilled actions were very poor. Generalized slowness, poverty of movements and loss of associative movements were among the main characteristics. . . . Tremor was not a major characteristic and, although 32 of the 47 had tremor, it was of mild or moderate degree. Fifteen of the patients did not have

tremor or any other involuntary movement at rest or during activity. . . .
In 19 patients, there was definite increased muscle tonus, rigidity, and
cogwheel rigidity but in 28 there was no appreciable rigidity although
their postures and faces suggested it should be severe. . . . A history of
mental slowness and poor memory was present in all patients and in
many this was the dominant clinical feature. . . . The mental picture was
organic and not of a functional, emotional or psychogenic type. There
was disorientation, memory impairment for recent and past events, and
difficulty in simple calculation. Depression was a common finding and
some had a history of hallucination. In the late stages patients became
apathetic, mute, immobile, lacked spontaneity, and finally fell into a
progressive vegetative state before infection terminated life.[30]

The Guam complex retained an enigmatic allure on a small group of neurological researchers for over half a century.

In 1994, neurologist and writer Oliver Sacks visited Guam to work with John Steele, a Canadian colleague who moved to the island in 1983, twenty years after his work on the identification of progressive supranuclear palsy—PSP, initially named Steele–Richardson–Olszewski syndrome. The narrative arc of what took place over the course of four decades, from 1961, is poignantly captured by Sacks as a disappointing detective story in which an initial intrigue, namely the Zimmerman finding, spurred a small committed group of neuroscientists to search for an explanation, only to find not only no answer but also the quasi-disappearance of the very object of inquiry. As Steele later wrote of the decline of the ALS–parkinsonism–dementia complex, "In 2004, motor neuron disease, once 100 times more common than elsewhere is rare, atypical parkinsonism is declining, and only dementia remains unusually common in elderly females."[31] What remained, as Sack's inimitable neuroanthropological inquiry made clear, was a series of disconfirmed and repostulated hypotheses about the illness, as well as the people, and families who live and die with this, or these, disease(s).

Sacks narrates the first encounter he had with a family with *lytico* and *bodig*, bringing to life Hirano and his colleagues' 1961 description:

> I was struck by Estella as soon as we entered the house, because she
> looked so much like one of my post-encephalic patients as she stood,
> statue-like, with one arm outstretched, her head tilted back, and an
> entranced look on her face. One could put her arms in any position,
> and they would be maintained like this, apparently effortlessly, for
> hours. Left alone, she would stand motionless, as if spellbound, star-
> ing blankly into space, drooling. But the moment I spoke to her, she

answered—appropriately, with wit; she was perfectly capable of lucid thought and speech, provided somebody started her going. . . . With Estella, specifically, there was the sense of calm, of her being in her own world, the sense of an achieved equilibrium both within her, and in relation to her family and community. . . . But it was very different for José, her husband: physiologically different, as a start—for he had the most intense jamming, clenching, locking parkinsonism, where muscle groups, rigid, fought against each other and jammed each movement at its inception. . . . José's sister, who lives with them, showed yet another form of the disease, one marked by a severe and progressive dementia. She was at first frightened by our presence—she had lunged at me, and tried to scratch me, when we first entered the house. She became angry, and perhaps jealous, as we talked to the others. . . . She was also quite aphasic, and very restless, given to bursts of screaming and giggling— but music calmed and cohered her to an amazing extent. This too had been discovered by the family.[32]

Their children were not worried. Everyone knew, by the mid-1990s when Sacks visited the island, that the younger generations would not get it. Between 1960 and the mid-1990s, a genetic cause was downplayed, although not completely ruled out; a viral postencephalatic hypothesis was not confirmed, although not ruled out. A lot of work and resources then went into two environmental hypotheses: one concerning the ingestion of cycad fruits, *fadang*, ground into a flour and baked, and the other concerning high levels of certain minerals in the soil and water around Umatac, a Chamorro village that in the decade between 1955 and 1965 had rates thirteen times that of the nearest neighboring village.[33]

What is crucial for my own purposes is that the etiological explanations systemically came up short and that histopathologically, the very nature of the object, the illness, was indeterminate. What had especially struck Steele about *lytico-bodig* "was the lack of uniformity, the variability and richness, the strangeness of its presentations, which seemed to him more akin to the range of postencephalitic syndromes seen in vast numbers after the encephalitis lethargica epidemic in the First World War."[34] Sacks narrates how Steele had taken him to his laboratory and given him three slides to observe under a microscope. The first slide: "'Substantia nigra,' I said. 'Many of the cells are pale and depigmented. There's a lot of glial reaction, and bits of loose pigment.' I shifted to a higher power, and saw a huge number of neurofibrillary tangles, densely staining, convoluted masses, harshly evident within the destroyed nerve cells."[35] The cortex, hypothalamus, and spinal cord were all the same, he reports, "full of tangles."

"So this is what lytico-bodig looks like," Sacks wrote.

Steele gave him another slide, and Sacks asked him whether all cases looked the same. Steele replied that in fact he was looking at postencephalitic parkinsonism, the disease that Sacks famously treated with L-DOPA in the 1960s, narrated in his first book *Awakenings*. "I haven't done much pathology since I was a resident, and I'm no expert but I can't tell them apart," Sacks said. Steele handed him a third set. Sacks told him he could not tell whether it was *lytico-bodig* or postencephalitic parkinsonism: "Neither. . . . This is my disease, progressive supranuclear palsy. In fact, it's from one of the original cases we described in 1963— even then we wondered about its similarity to post-encephalitic parkinsonism. And now we look at the Guam disease . . . and all three look virtually the same." The tangles he points out, are similar to those found in Alzheimer's. "Perhaps the tangles contain vital clues to the process of neurodegeneration, or perhaps they are relatively nonspecific neural reactions to disease—we don't know."[36]

That was in 1994.

1980–2005: Anatamo-Clinical Overlap between FTD and ALS

By 1980, despite the committed group of people in the Mariana Islands, it had become clear to many that the Guam complex was not going to unlock a secret that would account for three diseases that appeared to be configured together. To give just one example, already in 1968, a paper titled "Evolution simultanée d'une sclérose latérale amyotrophique, d'un syndrome parkinsonnien et d'une démence progressive: à Propos de deux observations anatomo-cliniques" ("The Simultaneous Development of Amyotrophic Lateral Sclerosis, Parkinsonism, and Progressive Dementia: Two Anatomo-Clinical Observations") described two cases that were characterized by the association of ALS with an extrapyramidal syndrome and progressive dementia. In the first case, the ALS was the initial symptom; in the second case, it was the extrapyramidal syndrome and progressive dementia that came on first: "After respective illnesses of two and three years' duration, the patients died from labio-glosso-laryngeal paralysis. The pathological findings were those usually observed in A.L.S. and in Parkinsonism—neuronal loss and gliosis in the substantia nigra with extracellular melanin, but without Lewy bodies or neurofibrillary changes. In spite of clinical similarities, the absence of these latter pathological findings did not allow us to regard these cases as being examples of the ALS–Parkinsonism–dementia complex seen on the island of Guam."[37] To make the point simply: two highly heterogeneous clinical presentations may show highly similar anatomopathological signs, and two highly homogeneous clinical presentations may show highly divergent histological hallmarks. The subsequent question is how and on what basis to make knowledge regarding the well-foundedness of an overlap when there is no identity between clinical presentation and molecular pathological findings.

Nevertheless, clinical and pathological work continued in parallel to the work on Guam, conducted by a few groups, mainly in France, and then in Sweden, England, and the United States, building a clinical and an anatomical picture of the occasional co-occurrence of dementia and ALS, specifying that the relevant "dementia" that appeared with ALS was of a Pick type, rather than an Alzheimer type.

The first step in advancing the work on the co-occurrence of ALS and Pick's, after the initial clinical cases noting their occurrence, beginning in 1932, was a paper from 1957, a fundamental paper in this history of frontotemporal dementia diagnosis, by Delay, Brion, and Escourolle, "Limits and Current Knowledge of Pick's Disease: Its Differential Diagnosis," which was the first paper to differentiate Pick's from Alzheimer's disease on both clinical and pathological grounds. As FTD expert Bruce L. Miller and colleagues wrote regarding the differential diagnosis, "Pick's disease was described to feature frontotemporal atrophy with sparing of the posterior lobes with histology revealing ballooned cells and cortical-sub-cortical gliosis. The clinical syndrome of Pick's disease showed increased behavioral alterations, lack of insight, and relative freedom from apraxia and agnosia. In contrast, Alzheimer's disease featured more diffuse cerebral atrophy and on histology showed neurofibrillary tangles and senile plaques. Clinically, Alzheimer's patients had symptoms of agnosia, apraxia and problems with spatial orientation."[38] A second important step was the subdivision in the mid-1970s of Pick's disease into three subtypes, with only one of them having the presence of Pick bodies.

For the initial part of the period that we are concerned with, roughly the decade between 1980 and 1990, the linking or rather the reexploration of a link that had been made periodically since 1932 was done on a case-by-case clinical basis, before larger cohort studies were later undertaken by groups in Lund and Manchester, and then subsequently San Francisco in the 2000s. In the 1980s, neurologists gathered case-by-case observations of the people they encountered who seemed to demonstrate both diseases: atypical ALS complicated by Pick's disease or Pick's complicated by ALS.

Four logical possibilities were explored by teams in France and in Japan, and the inquiry later intensified by the Manchester and Lund groups: the French asked (1) whether these are two separate illnesses, which happen to appear together; (2) whether it is ALS affecting areas outside the motor cortex; or (3) whether it is Pick's atypically attacking the motor cortex. The Japanese team by contrast posited a fourth possibility that their cases of "presenile dementia" of a non-Alzheimer's type co-occurring with ALS were a distinct disease entity. What is important to note is that none of the four logical possibilities were definitely ruled out, and in the place of hypothetico-deductive testing, what has been established is a spectrum that aims ultimately to classify on the basis of information extracted from two noncoincidental planes: a phenotypic plane and a genotypic plane.

Prior to the emergence of genetic discoveries about FTD, ALS, and ALS with FTD, it is worth reconstructing how researchers considered the overlap. In a 1980 paper titled "L'association maladie de Pick et sclérose latérale amyotrophique: Etude d'un cas anatomo-clinique et revue de la littérature" ("The Association of Pick's Disease and Amyotrophic Lateral Sclerosis: An Anatomical-Clinical Case Study and Review of the Literature"), S. Brion and colleagues reexamined a clinical case of Pick's dementia, secondarily complicated, according to clinical observation, with ALS, and they compared it with twelve similar cases from the literature, going back to Von Braunmuhl's 1932 observations. The authors consider the first three hypotheses (leaving aside the Japanese group's postulation of the possibility of a new disease entity). Against the hypothesis that such cases are the atypical start outside of the motor cortex of ALS, they cite the fact that there is no superficial spongiosis such as is seen generally in ALS with dementia in the frontal or temporal cortex or in pure ALS in the motor cortex. Hence, in these authors' view, there seems to be something specific about Pick's, which then leads to ALS symptoms. Furthermore, they write, "There are marked focal lesions, i.e. in uncus hippocampi, similar to that of Pick's disease."[39] Nevertheless, they suggest that even if the second hypothesis seems to be the best one, "there is actually no definite evidence for it."[40] They briefly review the clinical case:

> Mr. A, born 9th April 1905, a retired *Gaz de France* worker, was hospitalized on the 13th April 1964 for behavioral troubles that had been developing since 1960, and that were considered initially as consequent to his retirement. The troubles progressed with the appearance of insomnia, anxiety, inexplicable fears, and a progressive loss of memory, as a whole considered as depressive reaction to his retirement. Initially the subject underwent an amphetamine based treatment for obesity, which made him lose ten kilos, following which there were memory losses pertaining to recent events, an aboulia, an apragmatism, a loss of affectivity, and a progressive disinterest.[41]

It is important to note here the local specificity of the illness assemblage. As the anthropologist Laurence Tessier has demonstrated, one of the distinguishing features of how frontotemporal dementia is understood clinically in France is via judgments of loss of motivation, in contrast to the United States, where the symptomatology turns on a loss of "care" and a loss of "emotions": two contrastive anthropologies, or views of what makes brains "social."[42] The neurologists continue: "One year before hospitalization generalized fibrillations appeared and a loss of muscular force in the upper limbs. Since a few months, an amyotrophy appeared in both hands. . . . During the hospitalization in 1964, we find a global image [*tableau*] of dementia. . . . There is a large reduction in the stock of ideas, which makes it so that the subject is incapable of conversation. All that remains is stereotyped speech in which the subject repeats the same thing with a silly air."[43] The neurological exam showed the beginnings of bilateral grasping reflex, especially of Aran–Duchenne amyotrophy, touching the thenar and hypothenar eminences (the fleshy parts of the hands under the thumb and little finger); spontaneous fibrillations of the four limbs were noted; muscular force diminished in the two upper limbs; and the subject had an acute event on the October 29, 1965, with coma, and died suddenly twenty-four hours afterward. The total evolution of the illness was five years from the start of the psychic troubles and two years from the signs of ALS.

Brion and his colleagues comment that the clinical tableau is typical of Pick's, which is complicated secondarily by ALS. Two things jump out at the authors in terms of anatomy: one, how discrete the ALS lesions are, which are found only in the cervical region and in the cervicobulbar junction. The dorsal and lumbar lesions were minimal and localized in the anterior cornua, not in the lateral columns. The pyramidal tracts were practically untouched. Regarding the brain, the authors were struck by how discrete the Pick lesions were, evident only in the temporal lobe. The motor cortex showed ALS-type lesions.

In their comparison of the case with the literature, they note first that seven of the twelve previously published cases from the preceding four decades confirm Pick's as the primary illness. In the other cases, the illnesses are concomitant. Second, unlike for cases of "dementia *plus* ALS," for which there seems to be a strong familial character, "there have never been family forms known and described [of Pick's with ALS]. Familial forms of Pick's disease are known, family forms of ALS, but never familial forms of association of the two processes."[44] As we will see, this observation will be disconfirmed as the underlying biology of both ALS and FTD is explored, showing that within families who present with cases of ALS, cases of FTD, and cases of ALS-FTD, a mutation on chromosome 9 will be shown to be largely responsible.

Third, the comparison of known cases shows that the lesional intensity is variable and repartition is irregular. In the authors' case, as well as one other of the twelve reviewed, intense lesion was limited to the uncus (innermost part of the temporal lobe), while there were minimal lesions elsewhere, all being Pick-type lesions. The location of ALS lesions is also variable. "Are we dealing with an extension to the motor cortex of a cortical atrophic process?" the authors ask. The hypothesis could be valid if the lesion of the motor cortex is identical to that in the rest of the cortex, which is generally not the case, or if the lesion of the anterior cornua is reminiscent of that of primitive dementia, which is also not the case, since it is usually the type of lesion observed in ALS. The authors point out that in diseases like Creutzfeldt–Jakob, the lesions found in the medulla are similar to those found in the cortex. The authors do suggest that the requirement of lesional identity in the cortex and anterior cornua may not be necessary if the disease, as far as the anterior cornua is concerned, comes from transsynaptic degeneration. The hypothesis could also be valid if only the pyramidal tract were affected, which is not the case here, or if the cortical lesions were very intense, which is not usually the case.

Are we dealing with two independent afflictions? The late nineteenth-century question perdures. To this question, Brion and his colleagues replied, "yes," to the degree that the motor cortex lesion does not seem too different from classical ALS. What is striking is how, from a purely pathological point of view, nothing quite adds up. Of the three hypotheses put forward: "coincidence," they thought, is hardly likely given how rare each illness is by itself; the third hypothesis, the start of ALS lesions outside of the motor cortex, is purely speculative. The second hypothesis, extension of the atrophic process underlying the dementia, seems the most plausible, but there is not actual evidence for it, they conclude.

The biggest change to the consideration of the overlap occurred in 1988–1990 when Pick's disease was reconceptualized as part of a broader spectrum of dementias of a "frontal lobe type." These dementias came to be viewed not purely from a pathological point of view but from a broader clinical and anatomical set of observations, underpinned by imaging techniques. Whereas to count as Pick's disease, a brain had to have Pick bodies on autopsy, the new way of viewing frontotemporal dementia was in terms of the relevant pattern of dementia, in which "prominent personality change and conduct disorder in the context of well-preserved spatial localisation and navigational abilities differs from the "posterior" hemisphere dementia characteristic of Alzheimer's disease, in which spatial disability is an early feature and social graces remain well-preserved until late in the disease's course."[45] The importance of the reconceptualization of dementia of a frontal lobe type was that it considered the dementia primarily from the point of view of function and localization. Broadly speaking, David Neary and his colleagues in Manchester were adding to the understanding that when listening to the symptoms and the history of the dementia in question, most of the cases of motor neuron disease with dementia fit a frontal rather than a posterior dementia type.

The overlap was further tested in a pair of papers from the University of California, San Francisco (UCSF), in the early 2000s: thirty-six patients with a diagnosis of FTD with no known diagnosis of ALS or family history of ALS were clinically and electrophysiologically assessed for the presence of ALS at a clinic specializing in the diagnosis. Five of the thirty-six met criteria for a definite diagnosis of ALS, and two had EMG findings suggestive of denervation in one limb. An additional five patients had prominent fasciculations (visible, involuntary muscle twitching), and six other patients had trouble swallowing but all had normal results on EMG studies. The authors wrote, "For a variety of reasons, all of these earlier studies including our own probably underestimate the association between FTD and ALS. Patients with FTD and ALS tend to present first to an ALS center rather than to a memory disorders center. This is supported by our own work showing a 31% incidence of FTD symptoms in 100 patients with ALS presenting to the ALS Center at UCSF."[46] A year later, they tested in the other direction: a cohort of one hundred patients with ALS were tested with neuropsychological tools. The authors stated that "diminished word generation was found in one-third. Of the patients with abnormal word generation who agreed to further evaluation, nearly all were shown to meet research criteria for FTD. In addition, one-quarter of the patients with normal word generation who agreed to further evaluation met research criteria for FTD; these patients had new-onset personality changes. . . . This study suggests that frontal executive deficits are present in half of ALS patients, many of whom meet strict research criteria for FTD."[47] Up to 15 percent of FTD patients and up to 30 percent of patients with motor neuron disease experience overlap between the two syndromes.[48] The coexistence of two disorders may be underrecognized, as patients tend to present to either a neuromuscular disease clinic or a dementia clinic.

Without being able to go into detail about recent lines of inquiry, suffice it to say that the overlap story between FTD and ALS became richer in 2005, when researchers used ubiquitin immunohistochemistry to show that ALS, FTD-ALS, and FTD were related pathologically and fit on a histopathological spectrum.[49] The following year, TDP-43 was shown to be the major disease protein in the neuropathology of both tau-negative FTD, one class of FTD among many others, and ALS.[50] The last major biological discovery pertains to familial ALS and FTD overlaps, the finding of a hexanucleotide repeat expansion (C9ORF72) identified in families with multiple members presenting with a combined FTD/ALS phenotype, which for many neurologists is a crucial path for further investigation.

Past/Future: A Search for Integration

Although there has been some accumulation of knowledge about ALS, one of the striking things is its perennial character as an illness that is relatively well-identifiable and yet recalcitrant in terms of both nosology and treatment. Currently, there is no integrated biological account of the motor and cognitive presentations of ALS. The available knowledge indicates that motor neuron disease can onset in areas of the brain "concerned with the expression of thought, planning, personality and speech, all aspects of brain function that are strictly 'motor' in a wider sense."[51] As such, for some researchers, there is some support to the view that ALS pathogenesis is linked to the neocortical evolutionary development of the anterior motor brain. Researchers such as T. H. Bak and colleagues have used the phrase "what wires together, dies together" to point to the idea that "there may be discrete systems whose boundaries have a role in defining the expression of degenerative processes."[52] Thus, instead of seeing ALS as a disease of selective vulnerability of motor neurons, the link with FTD and knowledge of their overlap has oriented some researchers toward an "integrated" view of ALS as a "multisystem disease" that may proceed by way of systematic functional paths.

A neuroscientific model has thus been proposed by Bak and colleagues to integrate dementia diagnosis into motor neuron disease nosography. The cognitive issues associated with ALS have thus been proposed as constituting a fifth major clinical presentation of ALS, alongside bulbar, cervical, thoracic, and lumbosacral regions: "It follows the same rules of disease progression as other presentations, spreading contiguously from region to region, with a predominantly caudal direction. Accordingly, *dementia tends to precede other presentations and is often followed by bulbar symptoms.*"[53] Put prosaically: Wherever the illness starts, it tends to move downward from there. Hence, someone who has limb-onset ALS, according to the model, will not have severe bulbar issues subsequently, and someone who has bulbar onset will likely have subsequent limb issues. Likewise, if someone is going to have cognitive issues, they will have them first.

This kind of model is integrative in a proper neurological sense. But it is only a model of a heuristic and general sort. Clinical counterexamples abound. In *The Human Body in the Age of Catastrophe*, anthropologist Todd Meyers and historian Stefanos Geroulanos take as their object of study changes in medical thinking about trauma, bodily integration, and regulation at the turn of twentieth century.[54] Their study is wide-ranging and for my own purposes useful given their identification of a historical shift in neurological and physiological knowledge beginning just prior to World War I. Between 1900 and 1934, the anatomopathological vision of illness, focused on sites of death and lesions, was being rethought by way of a concern with how bodies were "integrated" and how specific bodies endeavored to ward off or else adapt and respond to the threat of disintegration. What is crucial for my own inquiry is that their identification of integration/disintegration as a conceptual and medical-practical concern for physicians dealing with different kinds of trauma, ramified by the experience of World War I, helps to clarify a shift in knowledge about ALS: what had been considered a "pure" muscular skeletal illness became understood as a neurodegenerative illness, affecting not only motor function but also cognitive, behavioral, and language functions, which required a way of conceptualizing the integration of degeneration. As Meyers and Geroulanos explain, the emergence of terms such as "homeostasis" and the physiological understanding of the "integrative action of the nervous system," to use Sherrington's precise title to his 1906 work, were solutions to a problem of how an organism maintains itself dynamically, internally, and externally and in the movement between the internal and external milieu of the organism. Previously, the integration of an organism had been taken up as simply an evolutionary effect. Physiologists, after 1906, wanted to know how integration operates, meaning that integration became a problem for thought and living and not only a fact "of life": "thanks to what stabilization processes did the organism actually hold together?" Answers to this question would focus on the interdependence of bodily systems.

The reverse side of the coin is the interdependence and the interconnections of breakdowns, of which the compound pathology FTD-ALS is an object lesson. In the contemporary ALS clinic, the overlap of ALS and cognitive issues is for the most part considered only in terms of ALS-FTD. As such, I leave the reader with a brief account of a diagnosis in which the nosological indetermination gives way to a "sense of certitude."

Coda: Peter

Dr. Blumen looks up the next patient on the day's list: "Okay, so we have Peter coming in at 10 A.M., he's suspected ALS FTD. That would be a good person for you to see Anthony, I think. He's a Christmas tree farmer."

"Yeah and he was specialized in this kind of dance, eurhythmy," Jillian, the occupational therapist, said.

"Oh yeah, what's that?" Dr. Blumen asked.

"I don't know. I think it's some kind of interpretive dance."

I intervened and said that it is a kind of spiritual pedagogic dance, within Steiner Waldorf pedagogy, a German late nineteenth-century educational practice. Dr. Blumen googles it and reads out the *Wikipedia* entry. "Great trivia! And we thought James had good trivia!! Look here's a video. Okay, so Peter: Advanced ALS with FTD. Significant weight loss. Two-year history of progressive arm weakness. Was physically active: Christmas tree farmer and eurhythmy teacher. Went from being able to walk about 3 miles max to 1 mile max in the space of a year. Swallowing issues. Wife and brother say he has become combative and argumentative. Has seen a neurologist. Father had Alzheimer's. Believes he will live twenty years. Family wants him to be DNR/DNI [do not resuscitate/do not intubate]. EMG was fairly recent. Imaging shows frontal abnormalities. Testing, if he would be willing, would be great."

The neurology resident has seen Peter this morning. Dr. Blumen wants to hear about his case before going in to see him. She had thought it was better that I go in to see him with her, because he is, in the physician's estimation, suspicious of Western medicine.

The resident: "So, sixty years old, two-year progression upper bilateral weakness, no lower motor weakness. He was a Christmas tree farmer, very manual work, ten hours a day chopping trees; he showed us a video of him doing it 2010 [the resident does the motion of hacking with both hands above his head]. In 2017 he noticed he couldn't do it as long. Summer 2018 he couldn't lift his arms above his head. He had difficulty feeding himself and bathing himself. Then he couldn't grip the steering wheel, and so had to stop driving. He doesn't feed himself anymore. His wife feeds him, has to cut up his food into small pieces. No BiPAP use [noninvasive breathing assistance]. Leg muscles, down from being able to walk three miles to one mile. Some dyspnea. He scored 24 (on the ALS functional rating scale); speech was three out of four ('detectable speech disturbance'). Can't teach eurhythmy any more, had to stop in 2017. He came to clinic because of the weakness but already the referral included an MRI that the referring doctor had requested and that showed 'cerebral volume loss with apparent frontotemporal predominance.' Mood-wise the family finds him argumentative, combative, easily irritable. He scored 8 out of 20 on the cognitive screen—not good. His wife scored him 8 out of 42 on the caregiver cognitive screen—really not good. He has difficulty swallowing. No medications. For family history, he said his father had 'mega Alzheimer's.' His father was very angry and irritable growing up. He used to whip him as a boy. Once Alzheimer's was diagnosed, he mellowed out, didn't recognize his grandchildren any more, he passed in his 80s."

"When did the whipping start?"

"I guess in his forties [father], since it was when he [Peter] was a boy. We saw him walk, he needs back support. Naming is intact for high-frequency words but not low frequency. Eyelid closure is full. Fingers are extended, can't do finger taps, but can do toe taps. He has sensitivity. I'm concerned about nutrition, swallowing, and breathing. He is slipping when he is sitting up."

"Has he fallen?"

"No, he is tripping."

"Falling is my threshold for wheelchair. Dr. Blumen concludes: EMG is concerning; MRI is concerning for FTD; for the lab workup, mimic labs, and a list for UMN (upper motor neuron) and LMN (lower motor neuron), for mimics, for example, West Nile virus."

We left the conference room to go to the board and met James the dietician, who has just come from seeing him.

"Very difficult: He's having to chew, regurgitate, make it into a paste, then swallow it again."

Several people grimaced and made a sound of slight revulsion—*uggggh*. James then relayed that Peter says it's a problem for eating but not so much for drinking, even though the same thing happens with drinking. He's at high risk of choking: "I brought up the feeding tube, and I said that it is a more a quality of life and not a quantity of life issue, given their insistence that he is DNR. His wife said she didn't know about it, and would bring it up with the other family members."

Dr. Blumen, the resident, and I went in to see him. Peter was sitting on his hands, sitting up, his back straight against the wall. Dr. Blumen examines him; she taps his arms and legs to see if he has any response. She asks him about his symptoms and specifically about swallowing. He replies that he has to chew it into a paste, to make it creamy. He has a bit of a stare, I think to myself.[55]

"Are you taking any medications or doing anything particular to manage your symptoms?"

"Vortex healing."

"Yeah, I've heard of that."

"And celery juice."

"Celery is very good for you. I feel comfortable based on what we know saying that you have ALS. Do you have an understanding of what that is? It's a progressive motor neuron illness. Here is a diagram. The behavior and mood changes are characteristic of frontotemporal dementia, which is connected to the ALS. I would like to refer you to the Memory Center, to get a confirmation of the frontotemporal dementia diagnosis."

Peter's wife asks about how the two illnesses are connected and Dr. Blumen explains that some people have just ALS and some just FTD, that some people have both, and that they are part of the same disorder.

"Do you know what causes it?" Peter's wife asked.

"No. That is what makes it so difficult to find effective therapies. There is a medication called riluzole, which we put everyone on as it does slow down the progression of the disease, and then there is another medication, which we will tell you about but before discussing it, we send you home with some information to read and then come back to discuss it, because it is involved, requiring a port to be put in. I'll just go and get you that information." Dr. Blumen leaves the room.

"You're from France?" Peter asks me.

"I'm a social scientist, my name is Anthony, I live in France but I'm English, nobody is perfect. I'm here for a year based with palliative care, looking at how people are cared for and care for themselves when they have been diagnosed with ALS."

"That sounds very vital."

Peter speaks slowly, not slurred speech, but with pauses in between the words. He says that he wrote a book about the heart field and threefold walking. He explained that threefold walking is a way of walking in harmonious conscious relationship to the earth.

Dr. Blumen came back in and brought the discussion back to Peter's illness. "To get back to Peter, here is some information you can take home about the second medication, Radicava, and we can put in the prescription starting now for the riluzole at your pharmacy, and we can also put in a request for a palliative care consult, which they do though telemedicine."

"Sounds great," he said.

"We'd like to see you again in three months."

"Sounds great."

Two weeks before Peter's appointment three months later, I looked him up on the appointment schedule and could not see him. I asked the clinical research coordinator to find out when he was going to be seen, and when she pulled up his file, it said that he was deceased. Peter was not seen at the Memory Center, and he did not do any genetic testing.

Part 2
CARE

The ALS team is waiting outside an auditorium in the medical school. First-year students have been listening to talks all day, learning about "interprofessional practice" and "interprofessional education." The coordinator of the day's program suggests to Dr. Blumen that the team should go really slowly through what they do, since many of the students may not have heard of ALS before and may feel embarrassed about asking such a basic question. At one time, shaming students for their ignorance was a pedagogical imperative. Today, students' ignorance is carefully assuaged. Most of the team is there: Dr. Blumen, Georgina the research coordinator, James the dietician, Pia the speech pathologist, Amanda the physical therapist, Jillian the occupational therapist, Margaret the social worker, and Moira, who is one of the respiratory therapists. Their invitation to talk to the students today is a mark of the recognition the team has earned, nationally and locally, as an exemplar of high-functioning interprofessional medical practice.

Before giving them the floor, the program coordinator sought to underscore for the students the importance of the team's work and their skill set. She did so, first of all, by naming an expectation about the kind of medical professionals the school aims to forge: the course organizer preemptively thanked the students "for the amazing work they are going to be doing, this year and beyond," in their "microsystems," which is to say the small groups in which students learn and practice within a frontline care delivery unit, "really improving the function of their microsystem, improving the lives of the teams they are going to work with, and improving the lives of their patients." The core theme for the week and, over the course of their entire medical school training, she said, is this theme of interprofessional education and interprofessional collaboration: "working toward our shared goals of improving patient outcomes" by way of five core principles of teamwork, she explained: shared goals; clear roles; effective communication skills, which leads to mutual trust; and measurable processes and outcomes, so as a team they can ask how they are doing.

By way of juxtaposition: she projected an image onto a screen and described what she was showing: "So this is a photo from the 1940s, this is sort of the vision of the early twentieth-century physician, obviously a white male, so he is on his own, he is walking from door to door, it is very reasonable to expect that he is carrying the entire extent of medical knowledge in his brain, and all the diagnostic and therapeutic armamentarium that he needs is right there in that little black bag. He works alone, he doesn't engage in shared decision-making because that concept doesn't exist, doesn't really engage in chronic disease management, because in the early twentieth century if you get a chronic disease you just . . . Die . . . [laughter from the students], because there is not really a lot of chronic disease management. So it's a nice picture, but I think we can all agree that it doesn't work in our modern health care environment. Just the sheer volume of medical knowledge and our diagnostic and therapeutic tools has exponentially expanded over the last century, and any doctor or any health care provider who thinks they can exist as an island or exist in a vacuum or practice in a vacuum is really misguided and doing a disservice to their patients."

The image projected was of Ernest Ceriani, the protagonist of a 1948 *Life Magazine* photo essay by W. Eugene Smith, a pioneer of the genre. In 1948, the American Medical Association was preoccupied with the future of general practitioners in the United States, as medical school graduates were encouraged to pursue specializations, no doubt for multiple reasons, among which, obviously, was money. Ceriani was nominated to instantiate the figure of the "country doctor," based as he was in rural Kremmling, Colorado.[1]

"Luckily we don't have to work alone," the program leader said, "and this is really the model of the twenty-first century of the collaborative health care provider. Recalling that we need to care not only for the patients but for the complex health care system that we exist within."

The theme of the 1948 photo essay, it must be underscored, was not only a reification of the heroic solitary medical doctor, walking around the countryside with the extent of medical science in his head and bag. The essay was also precisely about the exhausting loneliness of being a rural doctor, serving so many people across such a wide geography.

A second photo from Smith's series is poignant and worth contrasting with the one shown to the students. Ceriani is pictured after having performed a caesarean section during which both baby and mother died due to complications. His purposeful bearing in the image shown to the medical students, as he walked across the countryside with his medical bag, contrasts sharply with his disconsolate countenance shown in this other image: slumped on the kitchen counter, holding a teacup in an almost automatic fashion, his gaze faraway, the ash from his cigarette threatening to drown in his seemingly untouched coffee.

The two points can be kept in mind about the multidisciplinary team, separately and in their interconnection: not only that multiple providers, each with specific skill sets and areas of expertise, can optimize attention to the patient but that also being a team might be a way of sharing the burden of attending to an illness that, currently, nothing can stop from progressing.

I bear the two points in mind because it matters for care of ALS, not only the desire to provide the best available care but also the maintenance of that capacity to keep trying to provide the best possible care.

Dr. Blumen took the microphone and made this point openly: after a brief description of the disease and underscoring the fact that it is 100 percent fatal, she said that for her, it would be "too overwhelming and sad" if she didn't have the help of the interprofessional team and the knowledge that together they can provide patients with "an incredible quality of life as well as quantity of life. Being treated by a multidisciplinary team is the one treatment we have that prolongs life," she said.

Quality and quantity of life is the ratio at stake and at the very heart of multidisciplinary care, a ratio that requires a judgment of how to live with the illness and how to care for those with this illness.

The importance of this organizational form and this mode of mutual support can be emphasized by way of contrast with one available account, a disarmingly honest account, of a neurologist, who, after three decades of private general neurological practice, described his inability to shoulder the responsibility and weight of care alone. He left medicine after thirty years as a private practice neurologist, and his decision, he confesses, stemmed in large part from his experience with ALS.

Antoine Sénanque, the *nom de plume* of a Parisian physician, with an office in the sixth arrondissement, left behind his vocation shortly after publishing his first book, *Blouse* (*White Coat*), in 2006, a memoire about his medical experience of diagnosing and caring for those with neurological illness, and it is a reflection more broadly on the work of being a medical doctor. "Our profession is riding for a fall," he wrote. The mistake, in his judgment, is that people are confused about what medicine is, thinking that if only they had the right doctors, medicine would be fine.

> Everyone defends medicine. . . . It encounters only tolerance and admiration. Patients share the mistaken conviction that it is scientific, deserving of the same respect as physics, astronomy and mathematics. People respect science. Without it, no salvation. It's fascinating to see how people adore it. As though it has never disappointed.[2]

A double disappointment, then: medicine is not science, and science does not bring salvation.

For Sénanque, as a lone neurologist, he did not have the means to intervene on the disease progression, and he lost the desire to support those with illness when faced with a lack of salvation and a lack of progress:

> I broke with medicine thanks to the worst of illnesses: ALS. It tore me from my life as a doctor, without clemency, efficaciously . . . ALS affects a lot of people, it suffices to see one or two per month to have the impression that it's of a frequency equal to the flu. The suffering person remains present, coming back regularly in your thoughts, multiplying daily consultations. Two suffices to make you think that there is an epidemic. It's a real neurological illness: untreatable and fatal. A gradual melting of the muscles that often starts with weakness of an arm or a leg. It is insidious. A foot that stumbles, some cramps, a hand that begins to claw up. At the beginning it doesn't look like anything worrying, it's limited. The patient comes to see you without much ado, with some simple thoughts on the question: sciatica for the dropping foot, cervical spondylosis for the hand that is folding. He expects his own diagnosis to be confirmed, to be able to leave your office quickly with your blessing, and a prescription for some physio.
>
>   . . . I try to say as little as possible, to crumble the truth, without transforming it. I speak of motor illness of which we don't know the origin, of variable progression, the search for therapies for which we are waiting. They grasp the trouble. They ask more questions. I try to choose my words. . . .
>
>   For ALS, I didn't have a lot of words, surely not enough and less and less as the years went by. The patient of whom I am thinking . . . didn't hold my lack of words against me. He came to see me often, even though I didn't encourage it. I would have willingly referred him to a hospital, to be done with him. I had the feeling that he drained me. He knew this as well, I'm sure, but that didn't bother him. He didn't care about my

problems of tiredness, of psychological wear. I always managed to find a little progress in his muscular testing, a tendon that contracted a little better, a gain of a half centimeter on an atrophied thigh. It was hard because he was really getting worse and in a linear fashion. . . . He didn't believe for a second my reports about his progress, but I was serious about the things I did. . . . A little before his death I saw him a last time. He came with a book on the topic of his work. He was a landscape gardener; he designed gardens. I don't know why but the present stopped me from finding his little monthly progress. He didn't hold it against me. He could no longer walk at all. "It's worse." I never saw him again. That'll teach me.[3]

Although it was ultimately a young patient, Evelyn, a thirty-year-old mother, with intense pseudobulbar symptoms (uncontrollable laughter and/or crying), who finally brought about his exit from medicine, the story of the gardener is critical for two reasons: first, that the clinical presentation and medical lack are unspectacular, with Sénanque simply running out of other ways to say anything other than an observation that was plain to see, and second, that he attributed the patient's disengagement from him as caused by his failure to say anything other than that which was plain to see.

The kind of care Sénanque was providing is not the recommended approach in today's United States. In 2009, the American Academy of Neurology (AAN) reviewed available evidence concerning the management of patients with ALS and included in their recommendations a referral to a clinic with a multidisciplinary team so as to "optimize health care delivery and prolong survival."[4] Moreover, as their report stated, this care "may be considered to enhance quality of life."[5] The mainstay of ALS management is symptomatic treatment and palliative care. What I seek to trace is how this AAN recommendation became normative. More specifically, I want to show the norms of comportment, attitudes, and rationalities that came together under the banner of multidisciplinary care, in the United States, from their inception circa 1975, along with the progressive development of a series of technical solutions and interventions. These interventions were configured as a set of possible responses within a wider problem space, which itself needs to be outlined.

The problem space brought together a heterogeneous set of discordances pertaining to medical practice around disability, end-of-life care, and the obligations of medical practice to accompany those they cannot cure.

In the chapters that follow, I take up first the development of multidisciplinary care as a medium of practice, or apparatus, described through a set of technical supports that instantiate the emergent normative convention to aid patients to live as well as possible for as long as possible. The supports are means through which, on the one hand, the body is worked on, ameliorated to the degree possible, but then also become the means through which a patient, and those who support them, can ask themselves how and whether they want to continue, as well as how these means are adjusted to what end or ends.

MULTIDISCIPLINARY ALS CARE

When does living with a disease, with a tableau of symptoms, with a set of physical degenerative incapacities, turn into dying from an illness? And to the contrary, how can dying from a disease be turned into living with an illness and with disabilities? How is such a transformation possible?

The recent history of ALS, since 1970, is a case in point of such back-and-forth motion that disrupts what is otherwise, as we have seen already in the first chapter, a known and expected trajectory of illness, a degenerative slope toward death. The aim of this chapter is to lay out the norms and the technical practices, within the medical field, that underpin and orient how medical professionals grasp each of these gerunds, living with and dying from ALS within a medium of illness management, the ALS clinic. It endeavors to seize the set of problems specific to each technical intervention established for assisting patients and to ask how they are interconnected.

While the case of ALS is particular, changes in the management of ALS as an illness have been part of a much broader transformation of the threshold between living with illness (chronic health problems) and dying from illness over the past half-century. From roughly the mid-1970s, there was, in most advanced industrial states, a simultaneous separation of the practices oriented to living with illness from practices specifically oriented toward managing the dying process; such separation, however, was also accompanied by their interconnection, such that living with illness did not have to mean living as though already dead, while at the same time, there was an increasing preoccupation with how people actually died with chronic and terminal illnesses. From the mid-1970s, a constellation of problems in chronic illness management was made to intersect with problems of end-of-life care.

For researchers concerned with the management of chronic illness and ways of dying in the contemporary, the mid-1970s is an unavoidable touchstone, or historical marker.[1] The moment can be characterized in two ways: from a slightly longer-term point of view, it is possible to discern the emergence of "dying" as a preoccupation from roughly 1960 to 1980, across advanced industrial nations, which emerged in relation to technical advances and social changes. Within this broad period of change, it is possible to identify a more specific period from 1973 to 1978, one marked by changes in how hospital medicine in North America and Europe endeavored to find responses to this broad set of issues.

Put schematically, the twenty years from 1960 to 1980 saw (1) the emergence of the hospice movement;[2] (2) the conceptualization of death and dying as a problem of "acceptance"[3] and of working through the "awareness" of dying;[4] (3) the emergence of patients' rights movements and legislation, to manage the timing of the end of life;[5] (4) the relaunch of a "right to die" discourse and practice, which included a variety of legal and illegal practices of hastening death, including passive and active euthanasia, as well as practices of assisted suicide;[6] and (5) and, more specifically, during 1973–1978, the emergence of a change internal to hospital practice, with the establishment of the world's first hospital-based palliative care unit in 1973.[7]

Although the major institutional events emerged in North America and in the United Kingdom, the work of Claudine Herzlich, to give only the example of France,[8] reminds us that there is potentially a complex transnational history to be written of the emergence of "dying" as a social preoccupation in this twenty-year period, with 1975 as the critical pivot.

Herzlich's 1976 article "Le travail de la mort" ("The Work of Death") provides details of the fact that already in 1970 there were colloquia dedicated to issues of "Le médecin face à la mort" ("The Physician Facing Death") in France, and that in 1974, a roundtable discussion was dedicated to "Le droit à la mort" ("The Right to Die") at an international conference on "Biologie et Devenir de l'Homme" ("Biology and the Future of Mankind"). My focus on this turning point circa 1975 does not deny the importance of longer-term periodizations, such as the classic work of Philippe Ariès, in his book *Western Attitudes toward Death from the Middle Ages to the Present* or his expanded exploration of the same theme in *The Hour of Our Death* (1977). It rather insists on the fact that it is not by chance that Ariès produced such a reflection at that particular historical moment. The intellectual production was itself part of the conjuncture in which questions were being posed, for medical practitioners, patients, and academics, about the (plurality of) attitudes one could take toward the phenomenon of dying and the practical question of the institutional practices and settings required to be well oriented to the contemporary preoccupation with dying.

At the same time, it was not a conjuncture in which dying was the only concern. There was also at this very time the development of coordinated "multidisciplinary teams" for dealing with a range of medical situations: chronic and terminal illnesses, burns, geriatric care, and sexual assault, among others. While in the United States, a multidisciplinary team approach to hospital care of patients with multiple needs was developed at Veteran Affairs (VA) hospitals, after World War II, of particular note is the fact that in 1978, there was the development of a trial outpatient multidisciplinary ALS center.[9] I consider that circa 1978, with the development of a trial multidisciplinary ALS clinic, there was an interconnection of multiple novel practices that had been developed over the preceding decade. Such an endeavor was the result of the articulation of a set of concerns around both how to care for dying patients and how to support, in practice, people with chronic illnesses and disabilities.

Dying as a Problem: 1960–1975

The conceptualization of dying as a problem, and a problem of acceptance, as well as of working through awareness of dying, owed much to the field-opening work of Elisabeth Kübler-Ross, the Swiss American psychiatrist, who began her seminar on death and dying with students from the Chicago Theological Seminary in 1965. Held weekly at the University of Chicago, it provided the intellectual, experiential, and experimental setting from which her landmark work *On Death and Dying* was published in 1969. Kübler-Ross's work with her collaborators, chiefly a hospital chaplain, theological students, interested medical personnel, and, most crucially, people facing the end of life, created a space in which frank and serious discussions about dying were made possible within the hospital setting. What is so impressive and striking about the book is Kübler-Ross's desire to know the experience of these people and her often highly nuanced interpretations of what patients say and also of what happens, in terms of affect and gesture, between patient and family, when people talk about dying. She was able to document effects of these interpretations, such as the capacity for something painful to be said, a change in affect, and specific gestures of tenderness, enacted before it was too late.

A second node in the pathway through this problem space was the work of Cicely Saunders, nurse, social worker, and physician—best known today as the founder of the modern hospice movement. In 1967, Saunders, after over a decade of planning and preparation, opened St. Christopher's hospice in London, a watershed moment in the emergence of the modern hospice as an institution. One can speak not only of a preoccupation in multiple venues but also perhaps more specifically of a problematization of dying, in the sense that Michel Foucault gave to the term: a set of indeterminations and/or discordances around an object of thought and practice, indeterminations and discordances relative to which multiple possible responses, interventions, or possible solutions are proposed.[10]

The historian of medicine Michael Stolberg provides crucial details for grasping what is specific about the initial period from 1960 to 1970 in relation to a possible history of the problematization of dying in advanced industrial countries. Stolberg's research gives empirical substance to the sociological commonplace that with industrialization through the nineteenth century, and with the movement of people into urban areas, there was an increasing need for care of the sick, since people could decreasingly rely on family due to distance and breakdown in family ties. Moreover, advances in medical knowledge and the development of the hospital as an institution meant that people actually went to hospital with the hope of being treated and cured. As Stolberg points out, "The more hospitals came to be reserved for the curable sick, the less many of them had room for hopeless cases."[11]

The hospice movement was a response to this development, providing a space outside of the hospital for the dying. There was subsequently a response to this response, from within hospital practice: dying as a problem should not be outsourced, and there needed to be spaces and resources mobilized from within medical practice for those who could not be cured but who nevertheless could be cared for by physicians.

The very broad image that Stolberg provides us with is that from 1800 to 1970, people increasingly went to hospital to get better, and when it became clear they could not be cured, for the most part, unless they died quickly, the activity and responsibility of care for the dying was transferred elsewhere. These outside institutions for care of the dying began to appear from the mid-nineteenth century; they were often privately supported and had a religious tenor. Importantly, "the majority of nineteenth and twentieth-century homes for incurables were not primarily a refuge for terminal patients. Some patients suffered from palsies, rheumatism or arthritis and other chronic but usually non-life-threatening diseases. In this respect, there were no clear-cut distinctions between almshouses, nursing homes and homes for the infirm, all the more so as the importance of medical care in all of these institutions increased significantly."[12] In effect, the historical point of view shows that a paramedical set of venues for dealing with chronic illness and dying patients interwove medical and spiritual aims, increasingly finessing interventions of both physical and spiritual palliation. Herbert Snow's Brompton Cocktail (morphine, cocaine, and alcohol) was used outside the hospital in palliative settings from early on in the twentieth century, and yet, as already noted, it was not until 1973 that the world's first inpatient palliative care unit was set up, at the Royal Victoria Hospital in Montreal, as a response to a perceived need for the hospital venue to fully take up the mission of managing dying patients within its walls, a model of care provided by Saunders's hospice.

The year 1976 then saw, in Europe, the passing of the "Rights of the Sick and the Dying Resolution" at the European Council, which states that "the true interests of the sick are not always best served by a zealous application of the most modern techniques for prolonging life"; 1976 was also the year that Karen Ann Quinlan's parents won their appeal to the New Jersey Supreme Court to take their daughter off a life-sustaining respirator, a machine that was keeping the twenty-two-year-old alive after falling into a coma; 1978 was then the first year that a dedicated ALS outpatient clinic was organized in New York, initially on a trial basis to improve quality of symptom management and palliative care for patients.

The purpose of the above sketch is to provide a sense of the interconnection of events, practices, and problems at this particular moment: hospital medicine had taken back the challenge and responsibility for dying patients, had begun to conceptualize the need for improved coordination of symptom management and palliative care for people with chronic terminal conditions, and had started to wrestle, in practical terms, with requests from patients and families to have the right to refuse lifesaving treatment, as well as to actively seek measures to end life.

At the same time, multidisciplinary care for chronic and terminal illness, such as for ALS, emerged in the context of the rise to prominence of the disability rights movement. It is significant that the American Coalition of Citizens with Disabilities was founded in 1975 and came to national attention in 1977 with civil action to force the US government to implement section 504 of the Rehabilitation Act of 1973, guaranteeing protections for people with disabilities.

Each of these aspects has been treated separately in different literatures. Sketching them together allows me to give a sense of the conjuncture in which patients with ALS found themselves from the mid-1970s and in which the event of multidisciplinary care for ALS occurred. It is, moreover, a conjuncture whose broad contours are still in place today and in which a question appears: when faced with a diagnosis of a terminal illness and when faced with the experience of living with it, how do individuals orient themselves by the social and technical aspects of the supports that are put in place to try to help keep a person alive, as well as confronting a possible wish to manage or else know something about how death will occur?

From Withholding to Supporting: The Beginning of Multidisciplinary Care Circa 1975

Given such a configuration of problems and practices, it is not surprising that clinically based medical discourse on how best to organize and operationalize care for patients with ALS began to be published in the mid-1970s. However, it is important to note that prior to the normative encouragement of multidisciplinary care in the mid-1970s, symptom management to augment quality of life was oftentimes weighed against measures considered likely to prolong suffering. Some neurologists explicitly wished to avoid interventions such as gastrostomy for feeding tubes and tracheostomy for mechanical ventilation, so as not to increase quantity of life, implying that the physician knows in advance that the quality of a life could not or never be sufficient to warrant an increase in the duration of that life.

In other words, prior to the mid-1970s, there was a prevalent attitude among medical staff, with regards to patients with ALS, that favored restricting interventions to prevent the prolongation of suffering. The logic was something like the following: if this is the "worst of illnesses," as Sénanque wrote (in the first decade of the twenty-first century), better not to stick around too long with it. As a British consultant neurologist put it, in a publication in 1984 concerning how they could do better to care for people with ALS, "The ethical problems are considerable," he wrote, concerning not pursuing interventions such as feeding tube placement and mechanical ventilation, "but the profession's objective in the late stages of the disease is to minimise suffering and not simply to preserve life."[13] As the same neurologist wrote, "We have not thought it right to embark on measures likely to prolong distress."[14]

In contrast to such thinking, the linking of means and ends within multidisciplinary care for ALS, beginning in the second half of the 1970s, followed the "logical dictates" of the illness, as a distinct ethical orientation for the physician: "Care is logically dictated by the disease process, and thus a rational treatment program can be undertaken,"[15] US physician and ALS advocate Forbes Norris wrote.

The "logic of care," for Norris, thus followed the clinical presentation of the illness, and the principle of intervention was that symptom management *should* be provided to all people diagnosed with ALS and that every phase of degeneration would present unique challenges and opportunities for intervention, with the benefits weighed against harms: a ratio of quantity and quality judged at relevant moments and ultimately by the patient and their entourage.

The challenge, circa 1975, was the rational programming of care at each step of illness progression. Such a rational program, as I will show, has a formal character, leaving open the question of the substantive rationality of particular courses of action. It is crucial to underscore that such a way of thinking about ALS was in fact an intervention in the medical field in both the United States and beyond. To cite an example that will be discussed at length, the striking changes in ALS care in Japan during the 1970s are a case in point, providing a logical extension of the injunction to support an extension of the quantity of life by all available means.

The first outpatient clinic dedicated to care for patients with ALS in the United States was opened at Mount Sinai, New York, in 1978, on a trial basis, to assess the continued need for such a facility implementing a multidisciplinary approach.[16] The Mount Sinai group published a paper about their endeavor and early experience, in which they wished "to assess the feasibility of caring for the patient with amyotrophic lateral sclerosis (ALS) through an outpatient facility."[17] They evaluated and followed three hundred patients over a three-year period. In their terms, a multidisciplinary approach meant that "each member of the medical team would be aware of the patient's medical history during the progression of the disease, and could therefore be brought in with full awareness of what medical or therapeutic care might be required."[18] The team that was brought together in New York prefigured iterations of such team-based care across the country and then the globe over the next four decades and beyond.

Forbes Norris, who had begun publicly articulating the need for a change in attitude since the mid-1970s, concomitant with the experimental outpatient clinic in New York, argued in a 1985 paper that "these patients may . . . live many months and even many years, so withholding supportive and symptomatic treatments adds appreciably to the duration of suffering. On the other hand, providing such treatment often increases the sufferer's quality of life in the remaining time."[19] Norris and his colleagues took the occasion to make a judicious criticism of how this kind of chronic fatal illness is treated, under the specific conditions of US health care in 1985:

In the United States convalescent care is limited to a specific number of days per lifetime, as though chronic illness of longer duration were nonexistent. These are relatively new developments, and probably physicians earlier in this century were much more attuned to the possibilities of successful care through the administration of symptomatic treatments. Our example is the application of specific symptomatic treatments to the care of patients suffering from the motor neurone diseases, particularly amyotrophic lateral sclerosis. We emphasise the administration of treatments at home because of the importance of the home in the maintenance of morale, although a secondary gain from home treatment is a noticeable reduction in the cost of care.[20]

It is important to note with respect to this "secondary gain" that the reduction in cost noted is a reduction for the hospital and insurance systems, and thus it must be acknowledged that financial and other costs are transferred to the families, who must find the means to pay for and facilitate care, sums that are frequently considerable.

The multidisciplinary outpatient clinic became the apparatus through which home treatment is arranged and supported. It can be considered an apparatus, a series of arranged operations, to the degree that the clinic is a means to objectify disease progression in the individual and has the capacity to transform those who attend clinic: a change in medical status, a proposal for a new intervention, hard decisions about what interventions to pursue or not pursue, and so on.[21] This apparatus can also be understood as a medium of care.

The technical supports that the clinic makes available specify a logic of care, as Norris indicated. This logic is not only a sequence of conventions, although they are also conventional. These conventions of care must be taken up, rejected, or transformed as part of a form of life for the patients. Each person in the medium of care or in contact with the multiprofessional apparatus, which aims to help manage the illness, must ask for themselves how they wish to proceed as the illness progresses.

I have briefly described how a new norm for patient care, *to live as long as possible, as well as possible*, arose in a double context: interconnection of a set of problems around disability and end-of-life care, as well as the development of experiments in outpatient care teams. In chapter 4, I describe how technical supports/interventions are made available and how the clinical staff enact work around the norm of living as well as possible as long as possible.

In the remainder of this chapter, I focus on medical discourse about the technical supports invented over this half century, since 1970, relative to the normative concern with the ratio of quantity and quality. I take up four technical supports that concern the means of disease objectification, nourishment, breathing, and end-of-life care. Specifically, these supports consist of the development of rating scales of disease progression, feeding tube placement, forms of respiratory support and the correlate concerns about the anticipated time horizon of illness, and multiple technical supports for end-of-life care, including hospice care, and in several states in the United States, including California, since 2017, the possibility of "medical aid in dying."

For each of these technical interventions, I ask how medical practitioners have considered the reasoning underpinning the development of each type of support, leaving as a theme for later exploration how the use of such supports is considered by patients. Regarding the method that I followed, I selected these four technical supports on the basis of the significant place they occupy in clinical practice. Then for each support, I created a corpus of texts selected from medical journals, from 1970 to 2020, to grasp medical discourse about the function and role of these supports and their place within multidisciplinary care.

Technical Support 1: Rating Scales

Within the broad conceptualization of ALS as an illness, there is a basic tripartite distinction between ALS pathophysiology; the physical impairments consequent to disease progression, measured through clinical testing; and the disability that goes along with disease progression, reported by the patient and observed by others. This distinction, operative in medical discourse, broadly considers physical impairment as a particular form of medical objectification, with disability properly speaking being the subjective manner in which any given corporal impairment is lived. For example, a jaw jerk impairment, or tongue atrophy, is connected to but not identical with the physical lesion producing the incapacity, and both are connected to although distinct from the fact that a person has a reduced capacity to speak or swallow that they consider a problem.

Different people are able to make different adjustments (or not), compensate for the impairment, and recognize it or not. It is crucial to grasp that relative to the impairments and disabilities produced by the disease, the normative orientation that considers it necessary to support the patient through disease progression, an orientation argued for by Forbes Norris in 1975, was accompanied by a search for ways of measuring both disease progression and the impact of such progression: the impact on not only how the person experiences the illness but also what the progression indicates about rate of change, significance and degree of the change, and, importantly, the prognostic concern of the time left until death.

Multiple "rating scales" have been created for ALS since 1979, which show, in a very basic way, how the normative change in medical attitudes to care was accompanied and underpinned by technical developments in ways of knowing the illness and intervening on the bodies and environments of those suffering with it.

These rating scales have been used for three main ends: to track progression of disease in the individual, to compare groups of patients, and to evaluate clinical trials. They have differed in terms of how they each mix or separate impairments and disabilities. All of them have been subjected to internal criticisms from within the neurological specialty.

Mixing Up Impairment and Disability

Two early scales mixed together both measures of physical impairment, objectified through physicians' tools and the extent of disability, as reported by the patient. The Norris scale, the first ALS rating scale, was invented to track clinical changes after experimental treatment. Its limitations include assigning to bulbar function and respiration relative weights that are today considered inappropriate; it includes impairments that are now considered unnecessary from the point of view of measuring degeneration, such as bowel and bladder function (even though problems with these functions can be severely distressing), and crucially it combines self-reported functions, symptoms, and clinical signs, thus mixing impairments and disabilities.

A second scale, the Appel scale developed in 1982, aimed "to provide a quantitative estimate of the clinical status of the patient and of the disease progression," calculated as a total score, likewise designed to be useful for both clinical management and assessing clinical trials. The reasoning behind mixing together scores of impairment and disability in both Norris and Appel scales was to have a global vision of the degenerative process, with the principle aim being able to judge the efficacy of any therapy in terms of its ability to halt or disrupt that process.

As the Appel team wrote, regarding the development of their scale, they were primarily concerned with creating a scale that could judge the relative efficacy of therapies:

> Since there is no effective therapy, efforts are limited to the use of agents that provide modest benefits. To evaluate such agents, controlled trials are essential, but these may be particularly difficult, considering the variability both in the musculature involved and in the progression of disease. A patient may experience rapid deterioration in speech and swallowing function, and yet have minimal change in extremity strength, rendering strength tests meaningless in evaluating disease progression. In contrast, pulmonary function alone may be a less accurate guide in patients for whom extremity strength is compromised and bulbar function is spared. The published ALS rating scales do not document this variable presentation and progression in a quantitative way. The most widely used scoring system [at the time of writing], the Norris ALS Score, uses 34 items rated with values from 0 to 3, and the optimal score is 100. This system is difficult to calibrate and does not include tests of pulmonary function.[22]

Not including pulmonary function is significant: the respiratory score is extremely important for prognosis, and while there are several measures of respiratory function, the major metric is a respiratory score based on changes in forced vital capacity calculated as a percentage of a predicted value, according to a formula based on age, gender, and height.

The general problem with any rating scale is how to correlate a physical impairment with its significance for the life of the person living with it, in terms of its impact on how to live and how long the person has left to live.

A specific impairment consequent to pathology may occur early on in the disease, but the course over time of that impairment may be quite different from the change over time of the disability. Hand use is a good example, in which early impairment may not lead to severe disability until quite late, especially if people are creative with their solutions. A decrease in "x" points on a combined scale must somehow be correlated to both physical impairment and disability.

Moreover, one of the concerns for any ALS scale was the degree to which it is linear (i.e., that the value between any two consecutive points does not change). The Appel scale has been shown to be nonlinear during early and late stages of disease, meaning that a drop in points at these stages is equal to a larger or smaller change in function than the change correlated to the same drop in points in the middle phase of the disease.

Within the ALS medical community, it became clear that any effort to make a total judgment of impairment and disability over the course of the illness faced a problem of interpretation of changes. It is worth pointing out that the Appel scale managed the tension by making the score a product of clinical measurement and clinical judgment only. For example, whereas later scales rate disability based on what the patient reports, the Appel scale rates disability based on the clinician's judgment: for example, the bulbar score is determined not by the patient but by the clinical team, based on recommendations given at the clinic visit. Concretely: the patient may say they are taking a general diet, but for the Appel scale, if the ALS clinic team recommends that the patient should have only chopped or ground foods and thickened liquids, the patient then receives a grade indicating a problem with swallowing.[23]

Distinguishing Impairment and Disability

In contrast to the Norris and Appel scales, a pair of tests was developed in the early 1990s that assessed impairment and disability separately: the ACTS ALS evaluation tests impairment and the ALS Functional Rating Scale (ALSFRS) tests disability. Basically stated: the clinician is responsible for measuring the amount of impairment, and the patient is responsible for rating the degree of disability.

A revised ALS Functional Rating Scale (ALS-FRS-R) was created in 1999. It has become a standard tool for tracking clinical progression, and it is the primary outcome measure for contemporary clinical trials of therapies that aim to slow disease progression. The rate of change of the ALSFRS-R, or ALSFRS-R slope, has gained widespread acceptance as a prognostic indicator. Its strengths are its sensitivity to change, well correlated over the course of disease progression from beginning to end, with a more linear decrease than other tests and a good correlation with survival. The original category regarding "breathing" was replaced in the revised version by three categories: "dyspnea," "orthopnea," and "respiratory failure," making it more sensitive to change.

The use of the ALSFRS-R as a surrogate outcome measure for clinical trials has, however, been questioned, suggesting that it is less useful as a global total score and more pertinent as a "profile of mean scores from three different domains (bulbar, motor and respiratory functions)."[24] As Michael Swash has written of the functional rating scale, "The commonly used summed score of all 10 categories in the ALSFRS conceals details of change within individual categorical subsets, an inevitable problem given the different sites of onset and differing patterns of progression in the disease. These considerations imply that the ALSFRS Scale is multidimensional, consisting of *several independent variables*."[25] Interestingly, recent work has indicated that while the FRS does broadly correlate well with survival and seems to be more specific in the three subdomains, nevertheless, it should be noted that "respiratory subscores by themselves are not predictive of outcome."[26] The critical question thus remains how to judge change over time and change following possible treatment in an illness with such heterogeneous presentation and in which there is no clear correlation between pathology, impairment, and disability.

Using Scales in Trial Evaluations: Riluzole, Radicava, AMX0035

There are currently two drugs approved in the United States, by the FDA, as a disease-modifying treatment for ALS: riluzole was approved in 1995 and Radicava in 2017. Broadly speaking, after a new diagnosis, all patients at the clinic in which I conducted my inquiry are advised to begin riluzole. It is a benzothiazole originally used in a photographic developing solution and later as an industrial bleach. The legend that surrounds the development of riluzole as an ALS drug is that it was accidently screened in an in vitro assay of glutamate inhibition and found to be effective. First developed for use as an anticonvulsant, with increasing adherence by physicians to the theme of excitotoxicity in ALS pathophysiology, it was then tested in a clinical trial by the Meininger group at the Pitié-Salpetrière in France. Most people, however, patients, families, and physicians included, are clear about the limited benefits of the drug: it has been shown to increase survival by approximately two to three months, without demonstrable effects on quality of life. As Turner and colleagues state in their review of the two riluzole clinical trial papers in their *Landmark Papers in Neurology*, "Lack of subjective improvement, inability to quantify individual slowing of progression, and omission of quality of life measures from the trials, are commonly stated concerns by the significant number of neurologists who remain skeptical about the value of riluzole."[27]

The original clinical trial design was flawed in the view of multiple neurological researchers. Primary efficacy outcomes were prospectively defined as survival without tracheostomy and changes in functional status, using a modified Norris scale. Among other issues, British neurologist Ammar Al-Chalabi and colleagues wrote, "There is also concern that prolonging survival as disability worsens is futile."[28]

The approval of riluzole should be considered an ethical event to the degree that it raises the question of whether "any" treatment is better than no treatment. The approval of riluzole, which in effect responds positively to the question, provided the occasion for ALS physicians and researchers to criticize clinical trials that do not include both quantity and quality in their evaluation of the effect on life of any possible therapeutic molecule. As Miller and colleagues put it, "One of the greatest weaknesses of the earliest studies with riluzole was the lack of any quality of life data to support the limited benefit on survival. Adequate quality of life measures are now recommended for future phase III trials in MND [motor neurone disease]."[29]

In May 2017, the FDA granted a license for the second ever disease-modifying therapy for ALS, the drug edaravone, a free radical scavenger developed in the late 1980s as a treatment for stroke, licensed in Japan in 2015 as Radicut and called Radicava in the United States. Edaravone had been evaluated in a randomized placebo-controlled phase III study and showed no efficacy versus placebo.[30] For our purposes, what is important to note is that the efficacy primary end point was change in the revised ALS functional rating scale (ALSFRS-R) scores during a twenty-four-week treatment. The published results showed changes of −6.35 points (± 0.84) in the placebo group ($n=99$) and −5.70 points (± 0.85) in the edaravone group ($n=100$), with a difference of 0.65 ± 0.78 points ($p=0.411$).

While these results could have spelled failure for edaravone, the trial researchers engaged in a "hypothesis-driven post hoc" analysis, which "suggested an opportunity to demonstrate efficacy in a more narrowly defined patient population."[31] This population consisted of patients with earlier onset scoring 2 points or more on each ALSFRS-R item at screening, with forced vital capacity at least ≥80 percent and ALS duration less than two years: otherwise put, people who were earlier in disease progression. In the 2016 analysis, the mean change reported was -7.50 ± 0.66 (placebo) and -5.01 ± 0.64 (edaravone).[32] Importantly, Al-Chalabi and colleagues have written, "Previous studies have shown that most people with ALS decline by about 5.6 points over 6 months."[33] It is administered by infusion through a port, which has to be inserted into the body. The drug is administered once daily in a 60-mg dose over sixty minutes. Infusions are given for fourteen consecutive days in the first treatment cycle and for ten of the first fourteen days of each successive four-week treatment cycle: "Usage data indicated that 3007 ALS patients had been treated with Radicava as of 6 August 2018. Of these, an estimated 1006 patients discontinued treatment during that time. In aggregate, based on physician feedback, the reasons for discontinuation included disease progression, influence of the prescribing physician, insurance and financial burden, caregiver burden, clinical trials, and side effects."[34] As we will see in the next chapter, physicians at the clinic give information about the drug and say it's up to the patient whether to go on it or not. This attitude contrasts with the recommendation for riluzole, which is more declarative, possibly in part because its administration is less invasive, and the harms appear to minimal. Edaravone has not been approved in Europe.

I conclude the review of this first technical support with a case of difficulties in assessing what a molecule does for a patient: on September 3, 2020, the *New England Journal of Medicine* published trial data for a combination of sodium phenylbutyrate and taurursodiol. Participants were randomly assigned in a 2:1 ratio to receive sodium phenylbutyrate–taurursodiol (3 g of sodium phenylbutyrate and 1 g of taurursodiol, administered once a day for three weeks and then twice a day) or placebo. The primary outcome measure was the rate of decline in the total score on the ALSFRS-R through twenty-four weeks. Secondary outcomes were the rates of decline in isometric muscle strength, plasma phosphorylated axonal neurofilament H subunit levels, and slow vital capacity; the time to death, tracheostomy, or permanent ventilation; and hospitalization. The mean rate of change in the ALSFRS-R score was -1.24 points per month with the active drug and -1.66 points per month with placebo (difference, 0.42 points per month; 95% confidence interval, 0.03 to 0.81; $p = 0.03$). Secondary outcomes did not differ significantly between the two groups. Reports on the phase II trials have included a sober and balanced appraisal from Dr. Walter Koroshetz, director of the National Institute of Neurological Disorders and Stroke: "The data that we see here indicates there may be some beneficial effect but it doesn't look like what you'd call a home run."[35]

A significant further issue for continued use of FRSs as measures for therapeutic efficacy is recent work that has disrupted received wisdom that ALS disease progression is continuous. Bedlack et al. have shown that over six months, 16 to

25 percent of patients will show a stable ALSFRS-R score, an observation that may cause researchers to doubt the utility of using change in ALSFRS-R score as a way of evaluating clinical trials. As Bedlack et al. noted, plateaus in ALS progression lasting at least six months appear in about one out of six patients and could last even twelve months, eighteen months, or more in a smaller subgroup of patients.[36]

Technical Support 2: Feeding Tube

In the mid-1970s, when Forbes Norris and colleagues were arguing against withholding treatment, two kinds of technical/surgical intervention caused the most debate and concern within the medical community: mechanical ventilation and feeding tubes. Problems with breathing are typically accompanied by problems with swallowing, and virtually all patients with ALS develop dysphagia at some point during the course of the illness.

Normal swallowing is an act that requires strength and coordination supplied by a number of cranial nerves: the trigeminal cranial nerve (V) and the facial (VII), glossopharyngeal (IX), vagus (X), and the hypoglossal (XII) nerves, all of which are affected in patients with ALS.[37] Motor neuron loss leads in the early stages of disease to loss of lean body mass. As disease progresses, body fat, after an initial period of increase, begins to decrease in later phases of the illness. As Norris stated at the time, something that was well known for all who accompanied patients with ALS, "the immediate functional consequences of bulbar weakness are prolonged mealtimes and fatigue, which prematurely terminates meals. Of greater concern is the potential for insidious development of dehydration and suboptimal nutrition."[38] For Norris, the consequence of this situation was logical: "Initially, most difficulties are encountered in swallowing liquids, and, with progression, in swallowing solids. Attempts should be made later, or in severe instances, to stabilize the patient's weight."[39] Although not explicitly stated, the reason for waiting until later in the disease course and until the situation was "severe" may have been because the kinds of intervention available in the mid-1970s were not without risk and not easy to live with for patients— "Eventually most patients with involvement of the bulbar musculature require a nasogastric tube, a cricopharyngeal myotomy [a procedure in which the cricopharyngeus muscle, which makes a ring around the upper esophagus, is divided or cut across in order to break its grip] or a cervical esophagostomy [a stoma in the neck] to augment caloric intake."[40] These are serious interventions and ones that Norris and colleagues thought, nevertheless, appropriate under the right circumstances.

As late as 1984, Langton Hewer, a British neurologist, and colleagues gave a contrasting view to Norris's: "Bulbar problems are among the most distressing in motor neurone disease. These include dysphagia, choking, drooling, and dysarthria. We have not thought it right to embark on measures likely to prolong distress, and no patients were submitted to cricopharyngeal myotomy, gastrostomy, or tracheostomy and only one patient was fed by a nasogastric tube."[41]

Until 1985, patients with serious involvement of the bulbar musculature and who were cared for by teams who considered it appropriate to offer surgical interventions to augment quality of life were given the possibility of a nasogastric tube, a cricopharyngeal myotomy, or a cervical esophagostomy to augment caloric intake. The technical complexity of these interventions, their aesthetic aspects, and the complexity of use were key reasons why some physicians, patients, and families opted against such interventions, even when indicated. To a large degree, the surgical risk profile of feeding tubes was significantly reduced after the invention of percutaneous catheter gastrostomy and then percutaneous endoscopic gastrostomy (PEG) in 1984: a low-cost, relatively low-risk procedure whose technical management has been increasingly finessed over the past thirty-five years.

By the mid-1990s, "enteral nutritional therapy" was considered part of a correct management of patients with ALS and there has been an ever-increasing clinical experience and increasing data to show that early intervention, when the patient's breathing is good enough, poses little to no risk. Gastrostomy placement requires making an opening in the stomach wall in order to insert a plastic tube into the stomach. Liquid food can be fed through the tube, either manually with a syringe or through a motor-propelled drip. As Jeannette Pols and Sarah Limburg write,

> With PEG insertion, the patient has to swallow a scope that illuminates the stomach from within and the stomach wall is pierced from the inside out, thereby minimizing potential damage to blood vessels. PEG can only be performed when patients have sufficient lung capacity and do not depend on breathing devices. PEG placement is done by a specialist, the gastroenterologist, who in our study was associated with the ALS team and knew the patients from earlier consultations on ways of dealing with dysphagia (swallowing problems due to the weakness of the tongue and mastication muscles). When a patient does not meet the requirements for PEG but can lie on their back, the radiologist inserts the tube: radiologically inserted gastrostomy (RIG). With RIG insertion, the stomach is inflated with air and the stomach wall is pierced from the outside in. The diameter of the tube is smaller than

for PEG, fixed less stably, and the wound needs to be stitched, increasing the risk of infection.[42]

As such, the key issue today has become less of whether or not to propose a feeding tube and more a question of when is it the right time to do so in order to encourage use; as such, feeding tubes became a normative part of normal care, which may be refused for any number of reasons or excluded for medical reasons of contraindication.

Broadly speaking, the reason and justification for feeding tubes has been one of quality of life, but the argument about quality of life has always been accompanied by an interest in whether a feeding tube extends life. What is interesting about this is that it is a correlation that cuts two ways: on the one hand, some researchers and patients hope that they can show a positive correlation between survival and feeding tube use, while some patients and their family, as we saw with the Christmas tree farmer in chapter 2, hesitate to consider a tube not only because of issues to do with body image or acceptance of the illness but also because of fear that it will not only make them more comfortable but may in fact extend their life.

By 1998, the American Academy of Neurology practice parameters had stated that a feeding tube is recommended once there is progressive bulbar dysfunction. "Bulbar dysfunction and respiratory insufficiency appear and progress more or less simultaneously. This implies that delaying a PEG until dysphagia becomes symptomatically intolerable will be frequently associated with a low FVC, which may in turn increase the risk of performing the procedure."[43] As such, there is a broad orientation to getting patients to consider a PEG placement as early as possible in the disease progression.

The issue of the effect on survival of a feeding tube is debated in terms of evidence-based medicine: people who willingly and early on opt for PEG are looking for solutions for how to live with the illness and are able to adapt to the bodily and psychological troubles by intervening early. Such people are not common. PEG does stabilize weight in patients who experienced significant weight loss, but it is difficult to bring a not-yet experienced loss into a decision in the present.

It is important to note, however, that as concerns the American Academy of Neurology, there are currently no ALS-specific indications for feeding tubes, apart from the issue of compromised breathing. Since the precise effect on survival cannot be demonstrated, the chief argument in favor of feeding tube placement turns on quality of life and not quantity: in one of the few qualitative social science studies to take up ALS, Pols and Limburg studied what "quality of life" means for people who consider and accept a feeding tube during the progression of the disease. Their study was oriented by a basic pair of terms: the changes from having a feeding tube, both anticipated and effected, and the way those changes are valued by patients. They interviewed eleven people in a Dutch urban ALS outpatient clinic, eight living with a tube and three anticipating a tube, and they then also reinterviewed those who had been anticipating the tube once it had been placed.

The central issue brought up in their study was about timing: patients tended to delay tube placement as long as they could with a corresponding issue that many of the patients who opted (late) for tube placement died shortly afterward, posing the question of what the aim of the intervention really was for those patients. The researchers also narrate a very interesting example of a failed clinical trial at the same center, in which the research team wished to compare timing and outcomes between two groups: one in which the patients decide the timing and one in which the physician decides the timing. The trial could not get off the ground because patients refused to enroll, stating that they were not ready yet for a tube and didn't want to be in the group in which the physician decides for them. Broadly, Pols and Limburg learned a simple but important lesson from these interviews: that in order for a patient to accept a tube as a physical and aesthetic intervention, it has to be seen as solution to a problem that they actually experience; hence, there is a turning point, an event in time when a problem appears to which a tube can be a solution, to facilitate living in the way the person wishes to live.

Technical Support 3: Respiratory Support

Respiratory support for people with ALS is a critical element of multidisciplinary care and is both technically intricate and ethically charged: respiratory management decisions are closely tied to both survival time and the form of life that can be lived with ALS.

Respiratory failure is the main cause of death in people with ALS. The weakness of muscles used for breathing and coughing, as well as aspiration associated with bulbar involvement, conspires to produce pulmonary infection, sepsis, and respiratory failure. Crucially, this is what makes this area of support simultaneously technical and ethical: when respiratory failure and infection are prevented or treated, people with ALS can usually continue to live for additional years unless other medical problems occur. The body can be kept alive, on the condition that it is what the person chooses. It is important to note that while different kinds of mechanical ventilation have existed, technically, within medical care, long before 1975 (the invention of the iron lung for poliomyelitis being the classic example), long-term mechanical ventilation for people with ALS only began to be practiced after 1975, which is to say, only with the normative shift toward providing the means for people with ALS to live as long as possible, as well as possible.

The development of respiratory technical support has three aspects: the first is the emergence of long-term home mechanical ventilation, which was and usually still is chosen subsequent to an emergency event of respiratory failure, in which the patient is put on artificial ventilation and then must make a decision to live with a ventilator or not. Despite encouragement of best practices to gain patients' views on the issue of invasive mechanical ventilation in advance of any such events, it still frequently, in most cases, occurs subsequent to an emergency.

By making long-term mechanical ventilation at home a possibility, as a technical support, it became something that could be considered in advance and accepted or refused. The conditions under which it is possible must be reviewed. The second element is a brief comparative instance in which I describe the conditions under which, in Japan, from the 1970s until recently, most patients were put on tracheostomy ventilation and cared for full-time in the hospital and then subsequently, since 2000, increasingly at home. Third, I look at the changes over the past two decades, in which technical advances in noninvasive ventilation have led to positive effects on improving survival time and quality of life.

Making a Decision: Long-Term Ventilation at Home, or Not

An early case report from 1982 considering a series of six patients in Cleveland, Ohio, requiring long-term management of respiratory failure addressed a set of issues preceding respiratory failure, as well as problems deriving from hospitalization, planning for home care, and the psychological concerns that arise for patients using long-term mechanical ventilation. The series is of note to the degree that it shows how the authors considered character traits of the individual patient, disease profile, and family–environmental psychodynamics as pertinent elements in shaping how a patient can adapt, or not, to long-term mechanical ventilation.

A fifty-six-year-old "business executive" retired from work because of "widespread weakness," although at the time of his retirement, he had not been diagnosed with ALS. Respiratory failure developed fourteen months later, and he spent two years on nighttime ventilation, a period when he was still able to walk. From January 1980, he was on complete ventilator dependence:

He was able to cope with stressful situations by regarding them as challenges that needed to be overcome. Each time there were major decisions to be made as his ambulatory status deteriorated, he would approach the problem in an executive manner, make a decision, and seek the help of his wife, private physician, and other paramedical personnel to carry out his plans. The patient's wife accepted his being at home and spending time with her but expressed resentment that, as her husband's ambulatory status deteriorated, her primary responsibility became his care. Over time, she became more accepting, as their lifestyle changed very little because her husband had always anticipated that his retirement would be spent at home with her. She also expressed resentment toward her husband's tendency to give orders in an executive manner. She asked during one interview, "Is it normal for a wife to get angry with a husband who is sick?" He adapted to the situation. Although the patient is confined to a wheelchair with the ability to move only his fingers, he regards himself as being incapacitated rather than sick. When asked "What has it been like to be dependent upon a machine for your breathing?" without hesitating he responded, "It has been a friend. It has given me some extra years of life.[44]

Another patient was in his seventies, a retired roofer who went into respiratory failure after a direct laryngoscopy. A diagnosis of ALS was subsequently made when the patient could not be weaned within the first few days of ventilator support. After four months of hospitalization, he was weaned from mechanical ventilation and discharged to move in with his daughter. He needed supplemental oxygen, a tracheostomy (but not mechanical ventilation), and some help to get about. At the time of this first hospitalization, he had been concerned about who would care for his wife, who was undergoing coronary artery bypass surgery. "She did not appear to share the same concern for her husband, however," the case note states laconically.[45]

The report continues, describing him as having an attitude that alienated members of the family. His wife said simply that she could not care for him. Ten weeks later after discharge, he went to an emergency room (ER) with signs of septic shock: "The patient's family was advised that aggressive medical management was not appropriate, but the patient's son insisted that all efforts be expended, whereupon the man was transferred to our care [at the Cleveland Clinic]. When respiratory weaning became impossible, discussions about home care usually resulted in arguments between the siblings about how responsibility for their father's care would be shared. All the children insisted that they would not let their mother assume any of this responsibility. The patient himself recognized these problems and elected to remain in the hospital until he died four months later."[46] The lessons learned for this Cleveland team were that patients can adapt, in the full range of senses this term can include, and that technology has allowed a degree of mobility despite being dependent on a ventilator. "With proper training, family members can accomplish home care with little or no dependence upon medical or paramedical personnel," which is to say, technically they can do it, as long as they are able to commit to being at home full-time to care for the person, considering that even if some independent respiration is possible in the early stages, full dependence will follow. "From a psychological viewpoint, patients coped better when they viewed themselves as impaired or handicapped rather than ill with a terminal disease. Such an attitude also improved the abilities of family members to deal with periodic depressions."[47] An important observation, moreover, was that none of the patients realized the "full impact of their illness until sometime after ventilatory support was instituted."[48]

As the technology became available and clinical experience with long-term home ventilation increased, it became important for physicians to discuss with patients about what to do in a situation in which ventilator support is necessary. "If a patient decides in advance to avoid intubation or ventilator support after appropriate counseling then the family should plan what to do in an emergency and what medication to give to relieve respiratory distress."[49] It seems quite rare that a decision and plan is established in advance. Frequently, a respiratory event occurs, the person is rushed to the ER, and the person might be asked if they want to have their life saved.

Countercase: Japan

The model that emerged in the United States after the decade 1975–1985 contrasts doubly with reports from the United Kingdom and Japan. If the United Kingdom at that time had physicians willing to name their approach as one of withholding support for ethical reasons, Japan took up not only an alternative normative orientation with an attitude of encouraging symptom management on formal rational principles but also a substantive normative orientation that all patients should (must) have the maximum level of interventions, taken care of by the state with patients residing in hospitals. Balancing an imperative to care and an imperative to respect patient autonomy, although not uniquely American, appears in a specific form in the United States, against the backdrop of other clinical approaches that subscribe to an ethical choice to not preserve life, as well as against the backdrop of places that have longstanding traditions of intervening to sustain life at all costs, such as Japan.

A Japanese juridical framework from the 1970s concerning protections for people with chronic incurable illnesses efficiently made it mandatory to protect persons debilitated by ALS, rendering tracheostomy and mechanical ventilation normative and paid for by the state. Among these various forms of social security, it was making ventilators and home treatment free of charge within the health insurance system that most significantly increased the rate of ventilator use. The concept of *nambyō* (literally "difficult illness") was created by a set of legal articles in which these conditions are defined as follows: "(1) An illness whose cause is unknown, that is without an established method of treatment, and that poses significant risk of leaving sequelae; (2) An illness that, throughout its evolution, places a large burden on the family, not simply because of economic difficulties but because of the significant need for labor such as nursing care, or which imposes a substantial psychological burden" (*Nanbyō taisaku yōkō*).[50] Among these *nambyō*, a 123 particularly rare illnesses, from which recovery or return to society was difficult, were further defined as "designated illnesses." Forty-five of these illnesses, including ALS, were targeted for publicly funded medical care, with almost all treatment costs being subsidized by the government.

Since 2000, under financial pressure, as well as discussions of patient choice, invasive ventilator use has reduced, from close to 100 percent to about 30 percent. It must be noted that for those who do go on ventilation, it is illegal to take someone off it: "under Japanese law the use of a ventilator cannot be terminated once it is essential to a patient's survival, so to choose TIV [invasive ventilation] means to choose the possibility of entering a locked-in state."[51] As Yumiko Kawaguchi of ALS/MND Support Center Sakura (Tokyo) has written, herself a caregiver for a mother with ALS on TIV, "Many Japanese patients who currently use a ventilator say that their family members encouraged them to prolong their lives through ventilation. These family members have done so because patients are able to use long-term ventilation for only ¥1000 (around $11) per month, and can also access the latest communication devices and round the clock caregiver services in their homes at very low cost."[52] Kawaguchi describes the "extremely high quality of life" of people with ALS experiencing locked-in syndrome through their use of tracheostomy with invasive ventilation. She briefly tells the story of Ms. Hashimoto, born in 1953, who was diagnosed with ALS at the age of twenty-nine:

> Today the only part of her body she can move is the expression on her face. Until a few years ago, she was able to type emails with the middle toe of her left foot. In 2003, Ms. Hashimoto and I founded ALS/MND Support Center Sakura-kai, the NGO she runs today. The scope of this organization's activities continues to expand, not only in Tokyo but also

in other parts of Japan and even other countries . . . Ms. Hashimoto and other patients in Tokyo had established helper (caregiver) dispatching companies with capital from taxes redistributed through the welfare service for persons with disabilities, and were working as their employees. They demonstrated that even ALS patients on ventilators could work and contribute to society.[53]

The broad claim made by Kawaguchi, a well-positioned spokesperson for a specifically Japanese model of care, is that with the use of mechanical ventilation, people can go on living for decades, transforming a terminal illness into a chronic illness and set of disabilities. Around-the-clock care is needed, with someone watching over them at all times, even during nights, because of the risk of choking. Nevertheless, Kawaguchi makes the point that to view ALS as a "hopeless disease" is not the only judgment one can make about it. As has increasingly been recognized outside of Japan, if today for a minority of people, "invasive mechanical ventilation for patients who accept tracheotomy allows life prolongation and their QOL [quality of life] is not affected; medical teams should be aware of that."[54] It is unclear what it could possibly mean to say that a patient on invasive ventilation has not had their "quality of life" affected, regardless of what normative judgment one makes about the quality. The point nevertheless stands that some people do live this way, and some could live this way if the cost were borne and if the means were made available.

Noninvasive Ventilation as Standard of Care

Aside from whether and how a person might go on mechanical ventilation, prior to respiratory failure, a person might have respiratory issues requiring noninvasive ventilation (NIV). Although noninvasive ventilation tools have existed since the 1940s, chiefly in the context of treating acute respiratory failure, since the early 1990s, tools, practices, and knowledge have been forged in order to better treat chronic respiratory problems.[55] These tools and practices were created, moreover, in an institutional context of the creation of centers that focus on respiratory issues. For example, in 1987, there was the emergence of new clinical settings such as the "chronic respiratory care unit" at Bethesda Lutheran in Minnesota. These units were an alternative response to the kind of long-term hospitalization programs spearheaded in Japan, a less expensive model for providing chronic ventilator support.

Although supplemental oxygen was used clinically in a few hospitals in the 1920s, the first feasible means for sustaining life in patients who were unable to breathe for themselves came with the introduction of the tank ventilator (iron lung) at the end of that decade. The emergence of mechanical ventilation in its modern sense was spurred by the devastating polio epidemics of the 1950s, when experience in Denmark, and subsequently in the United States, demonstrated that tracheostomy and positive-pressure ventilation were lifesaving and long-term solutions.[56] With the development of intensive care units (ICUs) and as techniques for invasive mechanical ventilation were increasingly pursued, there was, however, an awareness of complications due to invasive ventilation, especially in acute settings like the ICU (first developed in the 1960s), where the ultimate aim is to ween patients off ventilators without damage to the lungs. As such, less aggressive noninvasive technologies were pursued to this end.

Already in the postwar period, physicians at Bellevue Hospital in New York began to study the use of intermittent positive inspiratory pressure via an anesthesia mask in the treatment of acute respiratory illness.[57] By the 1980s, there was increasing experience with long-term noninvasive positive pressure ventilation (NPPV) in cases other than care for polio, and then the first reports of use of NPPV in acute hypercapnic respiratory failure in chronic obstructive pulmonary disease (COPD) emerged. A technological development at this time included bilevel pressure-targeted ventilators (BiPAP). Unlike standard NPPV machines, which provide a constant singular pressure that can be difficult to breath out and against, a BiPAP machine has a prescribed pressure for inhalation (IPAP) and a lower pressure for exhalation (EPAP).

From the mid-1990s, the utility of BiPAP for patients with ALS became clear, and subsequent research was conducted on which patient profiles it would benefit, what the effects were on quality and quantity of life, and when to begin patients on BiPAP.[58] Although quality data have not been produced, one study from 2006 showed that survival with noninvasive ventilation was prolonged by seven months in patients without severe bulbar symptoms but not for those with severe bulbar symptoms. A yet to be demonstrated hypothesis is that noninvasive ventilation could delay deterioration of respiratory function. In terms of general positive effects, there is improvement in oxygen saturation and the apnea-hypopnea index, less daytime fatigue, and better sleep. Positive effects, however, do weaken over time.

Concerning when to suggest noninvasive ventilation use, most ALS specialists in the United States use forced vital capacity (FVC) measures as the prime indicator. By contrast, European ALS specialists report the occurrence of orthopnea and dyspnea as most important in prescribing noninvasive ventilation.

One of the main concerns in judging efficacy of the tool and to encourage compliance is comfort and ability to use it. The type of mask or device for air entering the lungs is crucial: full-face masks, nasal masks, and nasal pillows are three options, as well as the daytime "mouth-piece," which can provide a solution when there are issues with masks, such as discomfort. The importance of surveillance and correct-fitting equipment is underscored by the incidence of sleep apnea in patients with ALS, even for those with noninvasive ventilation.

As breathing deteriorates, a judgment has to be made about whether and when to transition to invasive ventilation, one that frequently, as discussed previously, follows on from a respiratory failure and subsequent intubation, unless the person has transitioned already to hospice care.

Technical Support 4: Hospice and End-of-Life Options

The fourth area of technical support, after scales for knowing something about the specificity of the illness for a given person, tube placement for supporting the sustenance and strength of the body, and breathing interventions to keep the body alive, is how to manage the end of life. Of course, other technologies are involved in care for people with ALS: communication devices, lifts and prostheses to aid mobility, home adaptations to facilitate everyday tasks such as dressing and washing, and so on. What is specific about the set of technical supports I have picked out is that they are techniques and technologies linked to how the medical field understands the development of the illness; hence, they are connected with the fundamental ratio of quantity of life in relation to quality of life, a ratio that changed the normative attitude of physicians in relation to this illness from the mid-1970s.

The normative intervention based on this ratio has a particularity that can be situated at a specific moment in medical care in the United States and can be distinguished from the Japanese position of focusing on quantity of life at all costs. Given this normative intervention, to live as well as possible, as long as possible, how is a judgment made about when to stop supporting quantity of life? As stated previously, there is a moment when a patient must decide whether to go on mechanical ventilation with tracheostomy, in order to carry on living, or refuse this option and to accept that death will follow. If the latter option is taken, it is important that the end of life is well managed since, as narrated previously, it is possible that a person may have a respiratory emergency event, thus ending up at the ER and then possibly being put on a ventilator. Or else, as narrated at the very start of the book, as with Michel, a respiratory event may lead to not being taken (back) to the ER and dying in difficult circumstances, something that could have been avoided with better palliative care.

Hospice as a practice, hospice as a place, and palliative care as a medical specialty emerged in the United States in a six-year period (1967–1973) and were very much intertwined. Over the past fifty years, the specific meanings of these terms have changed such that palliative care is now considered a medical specialty, within hospital medicine, dedicated to symptom management in cases where there are multiple kinds and complex layers of symptom control to deal with, as well as social and spiritual care issues. Palliative care, as a specialty, can be involved in patient management at any point in the course of an illness. By contrast, hospice, in the United States, is both a practice and a place dedicated to patient management in the last six months of life. A patient is eligible for "hospice" as both a place and a practice once they have a diagnosis of six months or less to live: "going on hospice" is thus an administrative categorization as well as a practical application of a set of interventions.

In the United States, hospital-based palliative care was relatively slow to start, beginning with the recruitment of T. Declan Walsh to establish a palliative medicine service at the Cleveland Clinic Cancer Center in 1987. To give an idea of the slowness of change, a noncancer outpatient palliative care clinic was established at one major hospital in Northern California, on a trial basis, only in 2015, even though the hospice movement inaugurated by Saunders and her colleagues took hold among US physicians, researchers, patient advocates, members of Congress, and members of the Executive Branch relatively early on. As David S. Greer and Vincent Mor narrated the situation in an article that appeared in the *Hastings Report* in 1985:

> Between 1980 and 1984 Brown University undertook an independent evaluation of hospice, as part of a nationwide research and demonstration project sponsored by the Health Care Financing Administration, the Robert Wood Johnson Foundation, and the John A. Hartford Foundation. The evaluation—known as the National Hospice Study (NHS)—grew out of a long-standing interest among members of the Executive and the Congress in the feasibility of introducing hospice as an option for Medicare reimbursement of terminal care. The study was designed to compare the costs and benefits of the hospice model of care (a multidisciplinary approach that stresses palliation rather than cure and incorporates the family and volunteers into the patient's physical care and psychological support)—with nonhospice terminal care, and to provide data for health policy makers regarding third-party funding options.[59]

In 1982, hence before the study was completed, Congress passed Public Law 97–248, the Tax Equity and Fiscal Responsibility Act (TEFRA), making hospice a federal program reimbursable under Medicare, the US national health insurance program (since 1965 for all people over age sixty-five regardless of income). Two years earlier, "a two-year demonstration project in which patients in certain hospices will have all of their expenses paid by Medicare and Medicaid was begun during the spring of 1980," showing an imperative from multiple stakeholders to intervene in end-of-life care and to find ways of aligning end-of-life care with the US health care and insurance payment system.[60]

To be eligible to elect hospice care under Medicare, an individual must be entitled to "Part A" of Medicare, the part that deals with inpatient hospital care, nursing home care, skilled nursing facility care, and home care, and the person must be certified as being terminally ill. An individual is considered terminally ill if the medical prognosis is that the individual's life expectancy is six months or less if the illness runs its normal course. For patients with ALS, this means having an FVC less than 30 percent of predicted. For the most part, when a patient "goes on hospice," they carry on living where they are currently living; hence, they do not move per se into "a hospice" (place). Inpatient hospices are rather rare as they are expensive to run. Where they do exist, they are designed for short-term stays to deal with symptoms that are hard to control or to give caregivers a rest. Importantly, in terms of the genesis of hospice in the United States, Greer and Mor write that "the advocates for TEFRA legislation . . . were primarily motivated by a strong desire to improve the life of the dying and their families, but elements of power and money also entered into the mix: nurses (mostly female) were anxious to throw off the yoke of domination by physicians (mostly male); entrepreneurs envisioned the development of profit-making hospice chains. The Medicare-supported system that emerged contained something for each of the hospice proponents."[61] Moreover, the National Hospice Study found that

> Patients in bedded hospices were somewhat less likely to report severe pain and had fewer symptoms than non-hospice patients. Their families expressed greater satisfaction with the care provided than the families of patients in home care hospices or conventional terminal care programs. Cost savings were substantial only in nonbedded hospices, however. While bedded hospices were less costly than conventional care, in the last weeks of life, the net cost difference in the last year of life was small. The NHS findings suggest that hospice is a viable alternative for families and patients facing a terminal prognosis, although the study does not demonstrate the dramatic superiority of hospice over conventional forms of terminal care. Since hospice costs were, in general, lower than the costs of conventional care, it appeared reasonable to finance hospice as an optional service under Medicare, and other third-party insurance plans.[62]

The timing of the report is important since, as mentioned earlier, the benefits of home care lauded by ALS physician Forbes Norris have as their correlate a shifting of cost onto families. As such, patients go "on hospice," a common current expression, not "into hospice," which means a set of visits per week by members of a hospice team. Going on hospice means giving up the right to reimbursement for any other kind of intervention designed to augment the quantity of life for the individual, including visits to the hospital. Hence, if the person was considering a feeding tube, for example, it would be important to have one put in before going "on hospice" (which in any event would be advised since it is recommended when FVC scores are above 50 percent of predicted). Having said this, patients can revoke their hospice status and then reenroll afterward.

Concerning technical supports for end-of-life care, a further one was added, which I will briefly describe since it will become important in the case material that follows in the next chapters: in 2016, in California, patients with a terminal illness with a six-month prognosis are able make a request for "medical aid in dying" to a physician, on condition that the person is an adult, that a physician has given a prognosis of less than six months to live, and that they are mentally and physically competent to complete the act. The law states that the medication must be ingested, which means going through the gastrointestinal tract, either orally or rectally (which is more complicated, but possible); hence, it cannot be self-administered through an intravenous tube set up by a third party (nurse or physician, for example).

Apparatus

Taken together, I consider rating scales, respiratory therapy feeding tubes, and end-of-life management as four elements that are configured together and which the patient, as an individual, must face, to ask themselves, in discussion with professionals, how they are going to create a ratio between quantity and quality of life.

Under the term "technical support," we can see the ways that medical professionals began to write about as well as practically organize support for people with ALS, starting from 1970, over the course of roughly a half-century (1970–2020). The focus in this book is on the United States, tracking a transformation in medical approaches to ALS in this particular context, a change principally characterized as a move away from a resigned attitude, one that was motivated by nonintervention so as not to cause unnecessary suffering (hence to do no harm) and not to prolong life with this illness. We can see, however, a shift toward a novel injunction (novel circa 1975) to live as well as possible, for as long as possible, via heterogeneous supports that subtended such an injunction.

Changes elsewhere in the world can also be traced back to the same historical moment, albeit with varying outcomes. The counterexample of Japan is an instance of a different way of taking up the same normative attitude toward living with ALS. With respect to the US medical milieu, based on published medical papers and reports, as well as neurological handbooks for the guidance of ALS management, my concern is with how medical professionals developed and discussed technical interventions for people, and into the bodies of people, with ALS; how neurological specialists began to objectify knowledge of disease progression in the individual patient; and the various options for management of the end of life with ALS.

ALS CLINIC

Based on observations from August 2019 to March 2020 in a multidisciplinary ALS clinic in Northern California, this chapter concerns a series of scenes that make visible the different practices of the professionals involved at the ALS clinic, the heterogeneity of their interventions, and the different aims and purposes of these interventions. To this end, I follow, broadly, the analytic strategy proposed by the sociologists Janine Barbot and Nicolas Dodier regarding how to study "the interaction between individuals and apparatuses (*dispositifs*)."[1] If the previous chapter laid out the development over the past fifty years of the core technical supports of the apparatus, in this chapter, I make a case for following Barbot and Dodier's approach by trying to comprehend the specific character of the "normative work" of clinical professionals within the clinical apparatus, when faced with the task of making use of these various technical supports. "Normative work," understood in their terms as the "evaluations, positive or negative, that people set out on states of affairs," becomes an observable, graspable level of inquiry through which to study how human beings interact with apparatuses (*dispositifs*).[2] As I explain, one of the difficulties (initially) of the fieldwork in ALS clinic was the relative absence of what could be called explicit normative work, explicit evaluations by clinical professionals about states of affairs for patients in the clinic: my initial difficulty in grasping what I was observing was that practices seemed to be purely technical. The aim of the chapter is nevertheless to argue that while explicit normative work was relatively absent, on further consideration, a crucial kind of implicit normative work was in fact at play for these professionals, the presence of which is crucial to grasp in order to understand the way that these professionals use the clinical apparatus to engage with patients with ALS.

The Discursive Implicit

Not saying something, or saying something indirectly, to another person in a given situation can have effects just as much as saying something explicitly to a person in a given situation. I am going to make a case for the importance of such a discursive implicit in the normative work of the practitioners in the ALS clinic. Following the argument of François Flahault in his *La parole intermédiaire*, building on the foundational work of Oswald Ducrot, the "discursive implicit" is a way, one among others, that individuals situate others in relation to themselves and vice versa.[3] The discursive implicit implies situating the other person by addressing them and not only communicating information about their "state."

Normative work in the clinic is thus not only characterized by moments of explicit evaluation or judgment about a patient's state but also constituted by an awareness about the constitutive relations between patients and clinical workers, a discursive and practical setting in which clinical workers are aware of ethical measures of "too much" and "too little" when it comes to evaluative statements, the affective part of ethics. It is through this awareness that a kind of speech that is "intermediary" is used. It is speech that is implicitly normative, a kind of speech that acts to situate both clinical worker and patient, the one in relation to the other, and each toward the object of discussion, which I argue is a version of the question that Flahault has underscored, namely, who I am for you and who you are for me, in this case relative to this illness.

The analysis of normative work in the clinic is an endeavor to try to grasp, at the same time, those moments of speech, in a given situation, in which explicit normative evaluations are made, the actual way in which explicit evaluations are expressed, and those moments of discretion, or of absence of evaluation, as indications (in both their presence and absence) of not only the professionals' endeavor to do their job of taking measurements, making recommendations, and discussing possible solutions to problems (i.e., *communicating information*) but also how those evaluations (or their absence) are part of the endeavor to manage both their own thoughts and feelings, their own orientation and attitude toward the illness, as well as the place that they occupy in relation to the patient and the place given to the patient whom they are encountering. The two instances that follow are situations in which one clinical worker considers that another clinical worker has been either excessive or deficient in the kind of normative work the other one engaged in.

Distance

Angela is a speech and language pathologist (SLP). She still works at the hospital, but only does a limited number of ALS clinics a year. According to those who know her, and worked with her, she stopped doing the regular ALS clinic because it was "emotionally too much" for her. She took work home with her, to put it in the words of her colleague, Pia. "You have to be thick-skinned to work this clinic." A sign of the difficulty, in Pia's view, was that Angela had very strong views about what patients should do, views about what would be good for them, views that she expressed to patients and their families. Angela apparently became very involved in the decisions patients had to make, which complicated her work and made it difficult to do the work. It became too much for her, Pia told me, and she stopped doing the regular ALS clinic. She did, however, continue doing the community clinic, in a small town 50 km away from the city, a satellite clinic that the team organizes once every three months. "There has to be a distance," Pia told me.

This small instance was told as a response to my own perplexity, expressed to Pia, about how the team did this work, week in, week out, keeping limits on what they could expect of themselves, as well as emotional and affective limits. In relation to Pia's answer, I was left with the question of how they establish, manage, and sustain what each clinical worker could judge as the right distance (hence also the right proximity).

I dreaded going to the clinic. The dread stemmed not from the encounters with people suffering from a difficult illness. Given the previous work I have done, illness, I like to tell myself, does not intimidate me; suffering, I know, is not pathological. Moreover, it is well known within neurology that patients with ALS are often described, as a patient group, as "genuinely pleasant," "pleasant and warm," and "unusually stoic and cheerful."[4] While I refuse to give credence to the idea that there is an "ALS personality," I mention this kind of statement because of the warm exchanges I had with people coming into the clinic, the pleasure I took in talking with them, the frequent moments of wonder at the fortitude of those I encountered, the humor, and the clear-eyed pathos of the situation that can never be entirely bracketed.

The few moments when the dread I felt in the clinic lifted were those moments, over those months, when I was given a place, a position from which I could hear what the person coming to the clinic had to say about their symptoms, about things going on in their lives, not only in the mode of technical report but precisely in the mode of narrating their experience, how they felt about things, expressed to me as someone situated in a position given by the patient or their family, in which I was something other than an appendage to the clinical apparatus, along with the various labels that would be given to me by others—a "French" social scientist (along with the confusion about my British accent), an "anthropologist" (along with the confusion as to what that meant), and a European "end-of-life specialist" wanting to know about ALS experiences in the United States (along with the confusion about whether I was a physician or psychologist), among other labels.

These moments of relief (from the anxious dread) were ones marked by narration, narratives addressed to me, situated in a position where I endeavored to hear someone telling me about their illness and how they were living with it.

That is to say, the dread and, more diffusely, the anxiety for me, as a non-clinical observer integrated into a clinical apparatus, lifted at moments when I could hear patients talk about their situation, and as such, they were moments when, through the explicit normative work of patients on how they are doing and living with the illness, I had, if not a "global" vision, at the very least a vision centered on "the person." This, I realized, is what I wanted to hear, which was to hear about what the other person wanted to say about how they were living with the illness.

By the same reasoning, I think that the dread I felt, particularly in the ALS clinic, stemmed from the occupation of a position (for the most part) in which my encounter with a person suffering with ALS was parameterized, limited, or constrained by what was said and done by the medical team: these were consultations with a series of specialists each responsible for the care of a body part or body function: speech, diet, respiration, physical and occupational therapy, and the medical doctor, responsible for diagnosis and medications.

The way that the clinic is set up has an effect of deterring evaluative statements about the individual as *a single entity*, to the degree that statements usually pertain to a partial aspect of the individual, notably of their body and specific symptoms, and not "Experience" taken as a whole, whatever that might mean. Even the structure of a clinic day mirrors this setup. The clinic begins with chart review of the day's patients. Patients are reviewed in the order that they will be seen; memories are refreshed as to who the person is, as well as what previous visits raised in terms of key issues, if there have been any; and specific questions that had been relayed to the nurse prior to the current visit are underscored. For any given patient, an assessment is made as to who needs to see the patient more urgently than others, and then that professional will try to get in to see that patient first.

Clinic workflow is managed on the board. It functions, in addition to its actual use and purpose, as an organizing matrix and can be read as a model of the clinical orientation. Without wanting to push the mathematical analogy too far, it is curious to note that there are moments of multiplication as well as division.

Broadly speaking, the people coming into the clinic, noted on the board with an initial at the beginning of a row, is "divided" by six columns referring to the different specialties. At the same time, several of the specialties often intervene together, multiplying their points of view, notably the registered dietician with the speech and language pathologist, and physical therapy with occupational therapy. As I will show at the end of this chapter, the one clinical member whose assessments have the capacity to make overarching evaluative statements that attribute "states" to the patient's situation is the physician (MD), becoming at times the "exponent" of the matrix.

What I found noteworthy is that there was no need, for example, at the end of the day, to come together to have a holistic view on what was decided or what issues came up for each patient. This knowledge is captured in the patient's electronic record ("chart"), and all members of the team have access to that information. It would not be noteworthy if it were only, or simply, a question of saving time or a question of efficiency. It is also that. I think, though, that there is also an underlying orientation, an attitude, that the team instantiates, in which their interventions, their work, is a matrix through which the body of the person coming into the clinic passes. How it all fits together for the individual, if it fits together, is not the purpose of their practice.

I think that it was the matrix, as the form of this medical consideration/intervention, its distance, and its moods, which was initially the source of dread for me and became an object of investigation. It is a distance that I think is produced by structured partiality, a set of built-in blind spots where no single clinical professional has a vision of the whole, and in my case, as one who did, to a degree, gain that vision of the ensemble, a nonclinical (anthropological) point of view on all the clinical points of view, these views did not (despite the relief I had felt of being occasionally addressed with narratives of "experience") add up to a view on the "person" or on their situation as a whole, something in any event that I had no clinical position or authority (or desire) to make any kinds of evaluation about, or to say anything about to the person concerned. Such partiality, or intentional limitedness, I think, can be understood as itself a kind of normative work.

Too Much or Not Enough

A second instance may help to underscore how, for those of us who are outsiders to the ALS clinic, this distance and the pathos of such distance, as well as this structured partiality, can be judged as problematic. It is a telling instance because it comes from someone whose clinical practice is typically oriented to consideration of "the person" as a whole, as an entity, and whose professional work, we will see, pertains typically to conducting explicit normative work with patients, so as to try to come to an understanding about their "state," taken as a whole, and in relation to their experience of suffering and oriented toward the horizon of death.

Timothy is a palliative care specialist at a clinic that works in tandem with the ALS clinic. He told me a story, the same story, more than once. He knows the ALS clinic well. As part of his familiarization with ALS as an illness and with how the ALS clinic works, he sat in on the consultations performed by the different members of the team. He is proximate to the clinic, professionally speaking, and yet his story expressed a concern that resonated with my own experience of the clinic.

Timothy was sitting in on a consultation while a patient was having her breathing examined. Her forced vital capacity was measured, which was said (aloud) to be in the twenties (20 percent of predicted forced vital capacity). The two respiratory therapists finished noting the values in the patient's records and then left. Timothy sat with the patient and her husband, as they waited for the next team member to come in. In his telling of the story, Timothy said to the patient that he was sorry and that it must have been really hard to have heard the numbers. What Timothy knew and what he anticipated—what he assumed— that the patient knew is the significance of a measurement under 30 percent, to wit, a life expectancy (statistically speaking) of less than six months. In Timothy's view, qua palliative care physician, the scene was problematic precisely because no *evaluation* of the value was made, no assessment, no attribution of an overall signification, and no affective addendum to the measurement, a lack that he felt obliged to fill in with his own evaluation: "that it must be very hard" (for her to have heard this).

To underscore a theme to which I will return, what Timothy was making quite explicit (although not "totally" explicit), at least in the way he was telling me the story, is a position for the patient and a position for himself relative to the position he made available for the patient: the position of the patient is one of a person facing a near-term horizon of death, a position of the dying person, and the position he is making available for himself is the one of a palliative care physician whose expertise is to accompany the dying. In his position and practice as a palliative care worker, Timothy noted this absence of evaluation, the absence of making these positions available in speech, and I surmise that in his story, it is constituted precisely as a problem to be remedied and to which palliative care is just such a remedy.

In what follows in this rest of this chapter, I present a sequence of scenes from the clinic that shows how normative work around the measurements, assessments, and considerations, rather than being *entirely* absent or lacking—as in Timothy's description—is to a degree present, albeit in a delicate relationship to evaluation, opening up the question of what kind of positions are made available for clinical workers and patients in the clinic.

The first instance is a direct return to Timothy's observation and his understanding of what was, in his view, lacking in the clinical encounter he narrated. The instance likewise concerns respiratory measures, and like the instance narrated by Timothy, there is no explicit evaluative work and certainly nothing in the register of compassion. However, I will argue, implicit and nuanced forms of normative work occur. Furthermore, the first instance underscores how an implicit evaluation that aimed at a limited or partial object, an element of a situation, had to be clarified so as to ensure that the recipients of the evaluation did not think that what was being implied was something *beyond* the evaluation of a limited and partial (technical) element of the situation, namely, an explicit evaluation of the person concerned and of his wife and, in this case, their domestic life.

How Does He Ask for Help?

Laura and Moira came into the cramped halogen-lit consulting room to work with Peter (from chapter 2), who had been diagnosed that morning with ALS and was suspected of also having frontotemporal dementia. Laura asked about how his cough strength is—he demonstrated by hocking up a lot of phlegm; she asked how he has been sleeping—"fine"; how his weight has been—he lost 29 lbs. in a year and a half; how many hours he sleeps as night—eight to nine hours; whether he feels rested when he wakes—he said yes. Laura then conducted the respiratory test.

Respiratory tests produce numbers that are sometimes invested with significance, including predictive significance about time to death, and also sometimes questioned as to their veracity, given how variable and arbitrary they can seem to be. A little description is necessary to put this point in context. "Getting respiratory" (i.e., having the respiratory team administer the tests) involves a respiratory therapist standing behind the person, with a very delicate combination of precision and just enough force, while holding around the patient's head and neck with one arm and hand, so as to press a mask onto the person's mouth. Instructions will have been given, such as "three breaths, in out, in out, in, then pause, then blow it out. You got that?" When it is the moment to "blow it out," the technician will invariably start shouting, "Blow, blow! Blow! *Blow*!! *Blow*!!!"

followed by something along the lines of "*all the way out*!!!!!" If the patient breathed in when they were supposed to breathe out or if the team thought that the person wasn't trying hard enough (a situation we will come to), then they might make a comment such as "try and remember this" or "I think you can do better than that."

In addition to remembering the instructions, which under the circumstances are not always easy to follow—the "circumstances" may include added layers of sound, information, and confusion such as translation requirements and, occasionally, cognitive decline—there is also the technical issue of whether the mask is sealed properly, as well as the variability of the time and day of the test, in addition to the fatigue and stress for the person concerned with respect to getting to the clinic on time, the stress of being in a small windowless room with harsh lights, and the pressure of having someone, basically, shouting at them, while doing something that is not easy and about which the person knows is potentially loaded with vital significance.

Laura explained to Peter and his wife Akiko that "there has been a decline in diaphragm and cough strength"—he measured 29 percent of predicted on the forced vital capacity test. She told Peter that he "should get a BiPAP" and "should wear it whilst sleeping at night." The reasoning for the injunction was then explained; "you're currently working with a third of lung capacity, so the machine should help you with sleep and to feel better during the day."

Peter, it should be noted, had not complained about sleep or about how he feels during the day.

"Wear it every night," Moira then repeated, firmly.

We have here in this scene not an evaluation but a value, a measurement, leading directly to an injunction, bypassing explicit evaluative work but including implicit evaluative work. To be clear, "you should get a BiPAP" actually means, when rendered explicit: the numbers demand and justify that the respiratory team should put in an order for a breathing machine with a company that will fulfill this clinical request.

Unlike the example with Timothy, the lack of evaluation was also a way of not locating Peter in a single, closed position, relative to the injunction consequent to the respiratory values (i.e., of not locating him in the position of a dying person). This effort not to lock Peter into a specific position, within speech, in the way he was spoken to, and the way he was spoken about, I will suggest, is not an accident or an effect of indifference—that is, it is *not* that he is *not someone for the team*, but rather the normative concern is to leave open the question of "who Peter is" in relation to the breathing needs made visible by the tests. The effort to leave open "who he is" in relation to these measurements is shown in what happens next. A technical question about which kind of mask/nasal device he should get when the machine is delivered to his home opened up a larger discussion of the couple's domestic situation.

Moira asked Peter whether he sleeps with his mouth open. He considered his answer, and while thinking, Moira cut to her point: "When respiratory comes to your house, you can see whether it's better to use just the nasal pillows [short little tubes that go up the nostrils] or the full mouth mask. Do you sleep in the same room?" Moira asked. Akiko said no. "How does he ask for help?" Moira then inquired.

Akiko told her that he hasn't needed help so far. Given this information, Moira shared her thought that she would "just do the nasal pillows, then." Laura told the couple that it is easier to call for help with only the nasal pillows (and not the full face mask) and to take them off if he is feeling nauseous. Peter had very limited use of his hands and arms. Moira then clarified her question by saying that it is going to be more difficult to talk when he is wearing the machine and then explained *that was why she was asking about the room.*

What I think this exchange shows is that despite not engaging in any kind of emotional work around the breathing measurements, which were objectively bad and indicate a statistical prognosis of less than six months (proven to be true in Peter's case), and without engaging in any explicit evaluation of the measurement, including significance about proximity to death, nevertheless, the respiratory therapists were involved in linking the measurements to the therapeutic injunction that a BiPAP machine is necessary, regardless of how Peter feels. More important, the discussion of the BiPAP machine led to an assessment of the home situation, without then exceeding the technical parameters of the technicians' domain: it is none of their business whether they sleep in the same room, except to know whether he is able to call for help should he need it, implying that there will likely be a need or demand for such help soon. This point is made implicitly without at the same time shutting him into the position of the helpless dying person.

What is important again is not that he might need help *in general* with respect to his overall set of symptoms but in relation to the very specific point that BiPAP use, especially at first, can be disagreeable, can make a person feel nauseous, and, for someone who has limited use of their hands and limited movement, is necessary to be able to call for help.

In sum, the technicians are willing and able to make a certain kind of assessment connected to the specific part of the body and the function they are concerned with, as well as specific recommendations or even injunctions made directly from the values and measurements, but the technicians do not make links from that specific function to evaluations that involve saying explicitly anything about the person, their life, and the horizon of their death.

This Is Really Upsetting

In the next scene, I contrast the previous efforts of the respiratory technicians to avoid evaluative work with a scene in which a medical student tries her hand at precisely such explicit evaluative work, which is to say, speech that aims at saying something about, or endeavors to qualify, how "the person is" in a global way. The scene demonstrates how this can be problematic.

I was introduced to Emily, a final-year medical student, whose chief clinical interests were in neurology and palliative care. Emily, Dr. Blumen, and I were in one of the small examination rooms, after having reviewed the day's charts with the team, waiting for the first patients to arrive. I was to sit in on a call with Mr. Barras, whose breathing was getting much worse and who would have to make a decision soon about whether or not to go on mechanical invasive ventilation. In the last chapter, we saw how the question of going on mechanical ventilation is closely tied to how long someone wishes to live with the illness, with the progression of incapacity, and how they conceive the end of life.

As we waited, Emily and Dr. Blumen discussed the difficulty of taking what they called a "spiritual history," elements of personal biography of a patient that may indicate what "spiritual needs" a person has, in relation to a given medical situation. Emily said that during a session with a palliative care chaplain on the topic of spiritual history taking, the chaplain had advised the medical students to ask the patient about what has brought the person strength during difficult times in the past. Dr. Blumen then suddenly realized that it was just past nine, so it was time to make the call. "Hi, Mr. Barras it's Dr. Blumen from ALS Clinic. I'm here with Emily Garrett, who you met last time. And Anthony Stavrianakis, a specialist in end-of-life issues." As Dr. Blumen finished the prefatory remark, a knock came at the door, asking her to sign some paperwork. "So lots of specialists here to help you and listen to you." Dr. Blumen put Mr. Barras on speakerphone and left the room.

Emily asked Mr. Barras how he was doing. It is getting harder for him to breathe, he told her, and yes, it is worse than the last time they met. Emily confirmed that it sounds like he is breathing harder. As for the headaches that he was getting before, he gets some pain behind his head, but it is not too bothersome—only when he tries to turn his head, he explained. He confirmed to Emily that he is feeling weaker, and when he sits in an armchair, it feels like it's blocking his diaphragm. In order to sit in a chair, he has to lean on a table.

"Have you been able to carry on cooking? I know how much you love that."

"Yes, I love that." Mr. Barras did not answer the question.

"What happened to the Trilogy?" Emily asked him about the noninvasive ventilator he was using.

"What?"

"What happened to the Trilogy?"

Mr. Barras told Emily that he has a new appointment with a pulmonologist, Dr. Douglas. Emily replied that she would like to talk to him about the tracheostomy.

"What?" He replied. "I can't really hear you."

"I wanted to talk to you about the tracheostomy."

"That's why I have the appointment with Dr. Douglas. On Tuesday."

Rebuffed in her efforts, Emily was resigned to telling Mr. Barras that she is glad he will get to see the pulmonary specialist.

Although rebuffed in her efforts to talk about the possibility of a tracheostomy, undeterred, Emily returned to her question about the machine. She asked, again, about what happened with the breathing machine. He told her that they came and took the chip and that he is not sure about the results. As far as he knows, they have not done the overnight oxygen readings yet either. He asked Emily whether she has the results. She looked on the computer, and after a moment told Mr. Barras that she couldn't see them. A ball is launched back into his court: she asked who would go with him to the pulmonary appointment. It will be hard, he said, but he will make it up there. Again, he did not take the invitation to say more, so Emily asked him directly about his family. He replied that everyone is doing great; that yes, indeed, his youngest daughter was about to start kindergarten, and that yes, she was very excited. He sighed and indicated his frustration: "What do we need to talk about?"

Emily replied that she wanted to talk through the decisions that he needs to consider and to see how things are going.

He told her that the generic version of riluzole felt different. Emily explained that they are not different, but if he felt different, then that is what matters to her. She then asked how long he used the breathing machine during the day. Two to three hours, he said. "Do you get outside with your daughters?" He does. "That's important to you." It is, he replied. "What else is important to you?" To keep working, to keep moving, he said. "To be active, but you got no choice," Mr. Barras told Emily.

"Right, being a hard worker is part of your identity," she said.

"But you know, given these changes that's happening to me," he began to say, then fell silent.

"What has brought you strength in the past when you have been in hard situations?" Emily asked.

"Mother Nature. I loved to go on hikes, walks, camping. I can't do any of that."

"Could you maybe bring nature into your home?"

"No." Mr. Barras said, flatly. "Why are we talking about this?"

The frustration and sadness in Mr. Barras's voice were clear. Emily looked at me with urgency and silently mouthed the words, "*Can-you-go-and-get-Dr-Blumen.*"

This example is one of the rare moments where someone in the ALS clinic tried to have a conversation linking the question of how the person is doing to an explicit question of "who" they are and the changes to personal identity that occur because of this illness, a linkage that was clearly connected to a "lesson" learned in palliative care training, which, at least on this occasion, didn't have the intended effect—to wit, opening up a conversation about how the patient could integrate the degenerative changes happening to his body to the desires and interests he has.

As made clear in the particular instance, such a discussion was not welcome, it was upsetting, and Dr. Blumen had to intervene in order to recalibrate the situation, which she did by going over the broad decision facing Mr. Barras and by clarifying some of the parameters of the decision, including the fact that if he were to decide to go on mechanical ventilation, then he would need full-time care. She answered his question as to what he would be able to do, physically, if he went on mechanical ventilation, with the reply, "as much as you can do now."

Importantly, Dr. Blumen did not specify that with time, what he "can do now" will change, such that while it is true that mechanical ventilation will not be more debilitating, it obviously will not stop disease progression either, such that eventually, as in the instances described in the previous chapter, at some point he could become locked in. Dr. Blumen's reply typified what could be called a kind of clinical presentism, not looking too far down the line since, on the one hand, not everything is known in advance and there are surprises, and on the other hand, what is known about typical disease progression is difficult to integrate into a present.

The effort by Emily to connect the technical question of choices about different kinds of intervention to the broad question of identity was a rare one, in my experience of the clinic. It was not the case that Emily was looking to make her own evaluative statements about the situation of Mr. Barras. She was rather seeking to constitute through discussion with him an assessment of how he was doing in relation to the "global" question of his identity.

Such work is in contrast to most clinical practice, which evaluates or measures how someone is doing with respect to the very specific technical competencies that each technical specialist has as a clinical worker and in relation to the available technical supports.

The scene with Peter aimed to show how implicit evaluations were recalibrated when they threatened to aim at an object beyond technical competency and when they verged on producing a restrictive position for Peter within the therapists' speech as to who he was for them, namely, a dying person who is going to need a lot of help. This implied position was then clarified by way of a restriction to a purely technical aspect that is within the respiratory therapists' competence: the possible need to take off the mask at night, a task that he would necessarily need help with because of his inability to use his arms.

The scene with Emily shows what could go wrong when a clinical worker explicitly aims at an object/objective beyond technical competency: namely, an explicit discussion of "who the person is" in relation to their illness.

In the next two scenes, first with Ginger and then with Poppy, I want simply to show how combinations of points of view qualify, or requalify, how situations are evaluated: in the first scene, what seems to be a situation that is "going well" from the point of view of speech and language pathology and diet is quickly recalibrated by respiratory as being problematic, and in the second scene, a situation that by all accounts is quite difficult from the point of view of physical and occupational therapy is recalibrated as going "pretty well" from the point of view of the social worker, as well as the MD.

Sound the Same?

Pia (speech and language) and James (dietician) went to get Ginger from the waiting room. She rolled into the room in her electric wheelchair. As she reversed into position, James made parking noises, the kind of "beep beep beep" you hear when large vehicles reverse. Everyone laughed. Ginger came with her husband Dick and her daughter Maggie. Ginger's ALS is "bulbar onset," which meant that at the time I met her, she had no capacity to produce recognizable speech and had some difficulty swallowing—hence, Pia and James wanted to see her first. Her weight was up by a pound and a half. James was pleased. He asked if she takes two cans twice a day. Dick suggested that they do accounts in milliliters. "400 by two is 800 ml. So that's a little over three cartons, just under the four aimed for," James stated.

"Four was too much; it upset the stomach," Dick said, losing the subject of the statement in the process ("*the* stomach").

Dick and Ginger decided to extend the time for gravity bag feeding, which helped. James asked for more details about diet. "Appetite?" Ginger made a motion with her hand. "So so," he, said in her place, even though everyone understood what the gesture meant. "Well, you're at low normal." Dick asked whether that meant they needed to give her more formula. James explained that they cannot increase volume per feed, but they can add a feeding.

This suggestion was met with a jovial cry of mock outrage from Dick: "It's difficult! She doesn't sit around the house. She has things to do: she goes to Costco, goes to Target, she works, she's active! She prices things for an antiques house!!"

The small room positively buzzed with exclamations and murmurs of active interest about Ginger's work. Dick continued, saying how Ginger does all kinds of stuff and that he even came home one day to find her on her hands and knees trying to do a load of laundry.

"We know you're a fall risk!" Pia chipped in, then taking the occasion to ask about how Ginger's swallowing was and in particular how she was doing with water. Her husband answered for her that she needs thickener, and Pia reminded everyone that water without thickener is less harmful if aspirated, to which there were nods and murmurs.

Ginger was writing on her board while the others talked.

James took a turn to ask whether Ginger had dry mouth at night. Their daughter answered that she has had dry mouth for years, even before ALS. She went to the Pine Street Clinic at USC (700 km south of where they live) to have it checked out. "Oh yeah," Pia remarked, "you've traveled for your dry mouth!"

As we talk, Ginger finished writing on her board: "NOT TOO MUCH SALIVA."

Her husband carried on the thread: "I give her atropine drops, she doesn't like them but I managed to give her one this morning." Although something of a non sequitur, he mentioned something else that happened that morning. "They delivered a cough assist machine and suction. We don't need them, but now we have them." Pia asked whether she is using the "mask" (BiPAP). Her daughter, in a playful tone, said that her mother is "noncompliant." Her husband confirmed that she uses the machine one to two hours a day. Ginger gestures with her two index fingers, making a box or square in the air. "She only likes to wear it while watching TV."

Pia turned intently to Ginger: "How are you finding the pace of conversations?" Ginger began to write. For a moment, a rare one, silence.

Ginger showed Pia her board. Pia read aloud, "PEOPLE ARE SO NICE TO WAIT FOR ME TO FINISH."

Her husband started talking again: "We had this whole setup, we went down to the Apple store in L.A., where her sister lives, and got set up with the devices as a way for them to talk, but she got tired of doing it."

Pia asked Ginger whether she prefers writing. "I WRITE THE PRICE," Ginger wrote on her board, referring to her work at the antiques house. "I'm sure that adds some suspense!!" Pia said, and finished her part by saying to Ginger that she (Ginger) seemed pretty satisfied with communication. There was some more animated conversation, and the little room was filled with laughter and some stories: about Ginger's book club and about the weekly letters she would send the whole family, "kind of like blogs before blogs." And then, out of the blue, a computer-generated voice, which we all then quickly realized came from Dick's phone: "*Hello my name is Ginger.*"

Pia took the occasion to say something about different software and models, but Dick was too busy goofing around. "*My nickname is Skates,*" the computer voice told us. Ginger waved off her husband with a beautiful gesture waving and wagging her finger as though to say, "Oh, stop it, silly." James and Pia then left.

The respiratory team came in and asked Ginger whether she received the equipment, both the BiPAP and the suction machine, that they had ordered. Their daughter tried the same joke about being noncompliant, and Moira shot her a very dry look in return: "They give you a period of ninety days, but if after ninety days you didn't use it for at least four hours a day, Medicare will stop paying for it. And it has to be four consecutive hours. Did you get a cough assist machine?" Yes, they did. "Using it?" Moira asked.

"Doesn't need it," Dick said assuredly, looking at Ginger.

Moira looked at Dick. Very calmly, she asked, "Ginger can you cough for me?" Ginger made a terrible screeching sound. "Now you cough," Moira said to Dick. He coughed. "Sound the same?"

Dick puffed up his chest up and tapped his pectoral muscles like a gorilla, "mine's stronger."

Moira did not find it funny at all. "Is it true she doesn't need it?" Moira asked.

Silence. Moira then explained why expectoration is crucial to avoid infection and the risk of choking.

"Will the breathing machine improve her natural breathing?" Dick asked. Moira explained that no, it won't, but at nighttime, breathing, for everyone, becomes shallower, and for Ginger, it becomes even shallower, leading to a drop in oxygen levels and fatigue. It can also help to stabilize diaphragm function, which may help to give her longer life expectancy.

Doing Pretty Good

"So next up is Poppy." Dr. Blumen read from her notes. We heard that she was last seen in the clinic three months previously, as is typical. We heard that she has BiPAP all night; she has a definite ALS diagnosis and was doing outpatient physical and occupational therapy. Dr. Blumen read from the chart, "She is hoping to get In-Home Supportive Services" (IHSS) and she confirmed that the clinic made the recommendation for IHSS.

IHSS is a government program that provides domestic, paramedical, and personal assistance services for people with disabilities so that they can live independently or maintain employment safely. The IHSS program provides an alternative to living in an institution for many people. As a bureaucratic organization, it is a highly complex and opaque set of mechanisms and programs. The number of hours and kinds of services that a person is eligible for depend on factors such as whether the service provider is a spouse or parent and whether the person receives full-scope Medi-Cal (the California branch of Medicaid, the federal program that helps with medical costs for some people with limited income and resources).

Poppy's chart stated that they have discussed a feeding tube already at the clinic, as well as a possible speech device evaluation, "but she's alone, so feeding tube might not work depending on whether she is able to get any more help in. We'll talk to her about that. Let's find out if she can afford a caregiver. She has no use of her hands. She's currently on four hours of care, which would not be enough. She has no family to support her. She comes in with a friend of hers. Respiratory measures were 60 [percent of predicted], which is okay compared to her FRS [functional rating scale] of 18." It should be kept in mind that less than 20 out of 42 on the FRS indicates "advanced disease"; hence, Poppy's disability has advanced more rapidly than her respiratory impairment, which means that she may live quite some time in a seriously disabled state.

Amanda and Jillian, the physical and occupational therapists, showed Poppy into the consultation room. She came, as usual, with her friend, Lilly, in her thirties, roughly half of Poppy's age. Dressed in pink, Poppy shuffled in with her walker and slowly took a seat. Lilly walked in, found a chair, tucked one leg underneath her, and absorbed herself in her telephone, while Amanda and Jillian asked Poppy questions.

Amanda, chipper as ever, asked "how everything is." Poppy said that things were difficult. Amanda offered a guess at what was difficult, "Moving around?" Poppy simply replied with the word "hands." When Poppy walked in, her fingers were clenched over such that she had to do a kind of pincer grip on her walker and push it with the palms of her hands. "Legs okay or weaker?" Weaker. She said that she was having balance problems. She has physical therapy once a week to help. Amanda asked whether she has gotten any stretches for her hands. "My muscles make it so that I can't hold anything well." Poppy demonstrated by picking up a cup between the base of two hands, fingers folded over. Jillian asked whether she could use utensils. Poppy said "sort of" and explained that she has some with the big handles made out of foam but loses most of what is on the spoon. Jillian asked Poppy whether she has any help. "A caretaker a few days a week, three days, and a live-in caretaker for every night." Amanda clarified the situation by saying, "So sometimes you're by yourself."

Amanda and Jillian continue the discussion by asking what the caregiver does and what specific day-to-day activities are challenging. Turning water on and off is particularly difficult. Jillian brings up the fact that last visit, they discussed turning the shower bench into a shower seat, which could help with washing. Poppy said that she was looking to move, because her apartment is on two floors. She has fallen twice in the past two weeks on the stairs. "Were you able to call someone?" Amanda asked.

"My live-in was there." "Are you the live-in?" Amanda asked Lilly. Lilly said no. "Are you family?" Lilly said no, again, and then said, "sort of," and then shrugged: "I guess I'm kind of like family."

Jillian asked if the live-in was able to get Poppy up, by herself, or if they had to call someone. The live-in was able to do it. Amanda and Jillian discussed a few more things with Poppy and then left.

The visit had named several issues with no clear solution, at this stage: falling on the stairs, which is serious; difficulties feeding herself; very limited use of her hands; and a question as to how to change the bathroom setup to make washing a little easier.

Margaret the social worker then came in. She knows both Poppy and Lilly well. "Any big changes?" Lilly and Poppy replied in tandem, "We got rid of Maria."

Lilly followed up saying, "But we haven't replaced her."

Margaret looked at her file. "I have here that you have a 185 IHSS hours a month. Do they meet your needs?"

Poppy said yes, and then said, almost by way of explanation, that in addition to the caregiver (Maria, up until firing her), she has a live-in friend who gets room and board, helps her to bed, and makes her coffee in the morning. "She's a retired person, I try not to ask too much."

Margaret got into a groove: "I'm thinking *emergencies*, Poppy. There must be times when you are alone?"

Lilly looked up from her telephone for a second to say that she's a bad friend, that she should be around more often. Poppy said back to her that Lilly has three kids and three businesses and then replied to Margaret saying that she has a button for emergencies.

"Who pays for it?" Margaret asked.

Poppy said that she's not sure. "On Aging? . . . Choice in aging? . . . A social worker told me about it."

A kind of banter back and forth was established between Margaret and Poppy, both serious and light. "I've never heard of anyone getting that for free. Do they check it?" Poppy said she is supposed to check in with them once a month.

"Do you need to move?" Margaret asked. Poppy explained about her falls. "You have section 8," Margaret said, referring to the government subsidy Poppy benefits from in order to pay for private rental accommodation for low-income households. "They don't move you?" Margaret asked. Poppy replied that she has to find a new place herself, since the government housing authority does not do that work for you, and she explained that it is hard to find section 8 rentals.

"And they don't do the deposit either," Poppy said.

Lilly, without looking up from her phone, nonchalantly said that she is in the process of buying a house, a one story in Antioch, not too far from Concord, that Poppy will live in. She should have closed already, but it is taking a bit longer than expected; then section 8 needs to come out to inspect it, "which will be fine, it's a beautiful place," she said, without much ado.

"That's a great solution to a serious problem," Margaret said. "What will happen to the live-in?" Deborah, the retired live-in friend, will go with her. Margaret said that she supposes section 8 will give the OK on a two bedroom.

"I want a three bedroom," Poppy replied. "One for me, one for the live-in, and one for all the equipment." Poppy doesn't want to have to live among all those machines.

"Well that's a stretch! Did they accept?"

"They just came and did the inspection," Lilly replied.

"Have you been in touch with the Association?" Margaret asked Lilly.

"They told me that with my income, there wasn't much they could do to help."

"The system is so corrupt. There's a ten-year waiting list to get on the wait list, which is a ten-year wait list. Unless you have a couple of hundred thousand to give, in which case you go to the front of the line. Are you getting more hours?"

"I'm fine with the hours," Poppy said. "I just need to find someone, now that Maria is gone."

"No one in Concord will do this [home care] for twelve dollars an hour. That'll be one of the good things about Antioch as well, there are people who will work," Lilly said.

Margaret asked whether the roommate could do it, and Lilly replied that she's on Supplemental Security Income (SSI), so she can't work.

"You could be the provider of record and then you subcontract, you pay the tax on it, then you pay the person in cash," Margaret said.

"I never thought of that. Watch out: He's writing all this down!" Lilly said pointing at me.

"People have been doing this for thirty years, no one's ever gone to prison. People often subcontract out to family members because of the language. *Laotians*. It would have to be someone from the family not working to do that work."

"Deborah is moody. Depressive. Always bitches. She won't do showers," Poppy said.

"Right, so if you find someone who can: it's not a fortune, we're talking $200 a month."

"With Maria, the language was a problem. She spoke Spanish and she used that . . . 'Oh I thought you said. . . .' Even Christine [another friend helping out] says I'm becoming a lot of work," Poppy said.

"Right, because it's not Alzheimer's," Margaret replied. "They're used to just putting people in front of the TV and looking at their phones. When there are people who have real needs, and who have a mind and can express themselves, they're not used to that. . . . You have had to struggle for everything," Margaret said.

"Everything's a struggle," Poppy said back.

"Good to see you, Poppy."

Dr. Blumen came in to see how Poppy is and how the day went. They discussed medications and some other symptom management strategies, mainly concerning nasal congestion.

Dr. Blumen was pleased. "You're doing pretty well," she says.

"It feels like it's going downhill fast."

"Trust me," Dr. Blumen said, "it can go a lot faster."

For Me, It's More Like a Year

At the end of Poppy's visit, there was a glimpse of the not uncommon occurrence in which the physician was willing to make a global assessment of how the person is doing. In my experience, such evaluative statements from the physician were made only about situations that were going quite well or better than expected. In no case did I observe a situation in which a global assessment was made that indicated a person was doing very badly, although, as we will see in the next chapter, the clinic physician would answer a direct question if a patient asked, for example, whether their illness was "late stage."

In this last scene, an encounter between a patient, Si Chang, and the clinical team, I have selected an uncommon occurrence that I think, despite its status as uncommon, speaks to the role of the physician and to the capacity of the physician to make evaluative statements distinct from any other member of the clinical team.

I do this to show that while the clinic really is a team endeavor and that together they constitute the objectifying matrix though which the body and functions of the individual patient are passed, drawing on implicit normative work but mainly avoiding explicit global evaluations, the physician is nevertheless a distinct exponent and authority within, and relative to, that matrix.

Ms. Chang has made it clear that for her clinic visit, she only wants to see the respiratory technicians and the physician. The team was aware of her exploration of the possibility of requesting medical aid in dying.

Ms. Chang had an air of fragile quietness about her as she sat, alone in the exam room, waiting for the respiratory therapists to set up their equipment. She looked pensive and sad.

"Any shortness of breath?" Yes. "On a scale of one to ten with ten being panic, how would you rate your shortness of breath?" Eight. Colette put a pulse clip on Ms. Chang's finger: saturation, 99 percent; heart, 74 percent. "Cough strength?" It's okay. "Can you cough for me?" Colette asked. "Stronger," Moira said. "Do you use cough assist?" Yes. "How many times a day?" Once. "Try and use it in the morning and the evening. How is your swallow?" Okay. "Solids?" Okay. "Liquids?" Sometimes. "Weight loss?" Si Chang said she doesn't know. Her gaze didn't leave the floor as the therapists asked her questions and as she replied. "Sleep at night?" One to two hours, she said. "How many times a night do you wake?" Maybe twelve times. "How much did you sleep last night?" One hour. "You nap during the day?" Often. Si Chang said that her body doesn't relax. "Baclofen? [muscle relaxant]." Yes. "Maybe they need to increase the dose. Mention that to the doctor. You're tired." Very. Yes. "Headache?" No. "Do you use the breathing machine all night?" Yes. "They increased the pressure by five on the cough assist machine, it's okay?" Yes. "The oximetry data shows the longest continuous desaturation is less than forty seconds; mean low of 90 percent, settings are okay. I don't know why you are waking so much."

The problem, to put it this way, is out of the bounds of their technical domain. Si Chang has had enough. She said her neck hurts and that she is uncomfortable. I found myself, interpolated into the situation, responding to her demand. I got up from my seat and looked in the cupboards, searching for a pillow. I found one and maladroitly placed it behind her head. She grimaced.

Colette and Moira did the respiratory tests. The first was 47 percent. Colette said the number aloud for Moira to note. The second test went right down to 32 percent. Colette detected a lack of effort on Si Chang's part and asked her to try harder. They did two more, which hovered in the low thirties. Moira made a comment that there was too much variability. Colette checked her breathing with a stethoscope. Diminished on both sides; crackles right lower. "I know you're interested in the End of Life Option Act," Colette said. "You need thirtieth percentile for that. Now you're on the cusp. In one month you will likely meet the criteria. Is the machine providing enough support?" she said it is, and Moira and Colette left the room.

Back at the board, Colette explained to Dr. Blumen what happened and says she suspects Ms. Chang was not making effort in order to be sure that her numbers were low. She says that she shouldn't have said her numbers out loud, because the second went way down.

Dr. Blumen went in to see her.

"I know one of the things you wanted to talk about is the prognosis: and I understand that you would like to make use of the End of Life Option Act. One of the things you should know is that the medication can go in through a feeding tube. You just have to be able to demonstrate some participation in the process. The goal is to prevent people getting the medication against their wishes, so as the long as the patient can articulate a choice. Because your symptoms started in 2017, people typically decline at the same rate. So we're not seeing rapid decline."

"I feel I am. My breathing is at thirty."

"We always take the best number, so that's forty-seven: so it is changing but not changing rapidly. You don't technically qualify for it now."

"My hands are paralyzed; my legs are paralyzed. . . . If I stopped using the breathing machines, my numbers would be lower."

"That is not our experience," Dr. Blumen said, "The breathing machine gives support, but it doesn't improve breathing. The other alternative is if you start hospice, they can give you sedation and then you can go to sleep without the mask, and you may die."

"The other physician here said the prognosis is six to nine months so I should qualify."

"For me it's more like a year. Legally you need FVC of less than 30 percent. We have been able to get hospice without 30 percent before . . . if I say the patient does not want PEG and feeding tube, we might be able to start that."

"It's difficult to come here," Si Chang says.

"You don't have to come here. You can do your breathing tests at a pulmonary testing lab, and you would get hospice care at home."

"When can I do another breathing test?"

"Whenever you like, although maybe not before another month."

"I have a letter from a psychiatrist."

"When from?"

"Last December.

"That's almost a year . . . better if Georgina does a depression test."

"I don't qualify yet?"

"That's right. But you can qualify for hospice."

"I might go abroad," Si Chang says, implying that she might go abroad in order to do an assisted suicide.

"I want to make sure you hear what I am saying: if you go to hospice, they can give you sedating medication and you might die. We can also test your breathing, and we can prepare the documents for when you qualify for the End of Life Options Act."

"I'm not sure my breathing is bad enough for that to work. What FVC numbers mean that it works? [i.e., to go to sleep without the mask on and then to die]"

"It's hard to say: that's why also the length of the illness is the other important factor: since you've been living with it already for two years. Would you like to start hospice?"

Si Chang said yes.

PALLIATIVE CARE CLINIC

The outpatient (noncancer) palliative care provided at this medical center in Northern California is distinct from other symptom management services for cancer, as well as being detached organizationally from inpatient palliative care and pediatric palliative care, and it is distinct from a hyperspecialized palliative care clinic for Parkinson's spectrum disorders. It is worth underscoring the extent to which, historically, the first forty years of institutionalized palliative care, broadly, in both the United States and globally, has been tied to the needs of patients with cancer, as well as the effects and limits of cancer treatment, in the context of inpatient care within hospices and hospitals. The very recent emergence of a noncancer palliative care service at this particular medical center, circa 2016, was primarily a response to a recognition of a sought-after clinical encounter that was lacking in the ALS clinic. This outpatient palliative care clinic actually started within the ALS clinic, whose work was described in the previous chapter, and initially attended only by patients with ALS.

By 2019, with a widening of scope concerning which patients could be seen at the clinic and an opening toward all noncancer illnesses, nevertheless, at this time, still a quarter of the clinic's patients were those diagnosed with ALS. It is today a setting that is both distinct from the ALS clinic and yet connected to it. It is distinct insofar as it is an independent group centered on a trio of staff members, namely, a nurse, a social worker, and a chaplain, with a rotating group of physicians completing the team. They see nonhospitalized patients, either in person at the clinic or by "telemedicine" through videoconference technology. It is distinct and connected insofar as it takes up the "overflow" (to use Michel Callon's broad term for exploring externalities) from the manner in which the ALS clinic organizes work and the manner in which the clinical matrix of work constitutes its object of attention, how it "frames" the human being coming to the clinic (to use Callon's paired term).[1] To put it pointedly, the previous chapter endeavored to show how the framing of the human being in the ALS clinic is one in which personhood, in the sense of making overarching evaluations of who the person is in relation to the illness, is, for the most part, bracketed. I considered this bracketing as both a technical and an ethical practice of suspension, a suspension by the clinical worker of a possible demand for patients (and for themselves) to answer the question of "who they are" in relation to this illness.

Nevertheless, in terms of multidisciplinary medical care for ALS, the ALS clinic refers patients to the palliative care team once a question of identity or personhood is raised explicitly by patients in the ALS clinic. This question may be related to concerns about the horizon of death, as considered by the patient or the physician.

That is to say, in addition to moments when a demand is raised from, and on the side of, the patient, there is also the possibility that the physician makes an evaluative claim that the patient *should* (hence in a register of explicit normative work) make an appointment with palliative care.

As such, we can now say that in addition to *bracketing* "personhood," the ALS clinic produces an externality in which questions of personhood can be taken up by this other medical apparatus. Palliative care clinic is thus a medium for taking up and taking on this externality, attending to both medical needs, as evaluated by the medical staff, as well as addressing the demands of those who are experiencing the corporeal, affective, and relational changes brought on through neurological degeneration characteristic of this illness.

Only through description and analysis will I be able to say more about how a human being appears in a palliative care clinic: for example, whether or how it appears as an "individual," as a "person," as a "self," as a "relation," or as a "subject," which is to say, a position in and effect of language. Other occasions for referral from ALS to a palliative care clinic include moments when there is a question of what *they want* (to do, to have done to them), in relation to this horizon of death.

Sometimes the ALS clinic will actively suggest that patients go to meet the palliative care team if either the objective evaluation of the disease process indicates that they will soon die (hence a question of a medical evaluation organizing the management of the end-of-life period of illness, rather than a demand from the patient) or the physician in the ALS clinic considers that these questions—questions linked to a horizon of death or to identity—are causing suffering by not being addressed. In any event, it is the (normative) work of the palliative care team to deal with the twin externalized poles of (to state it briefly) *identity* and the *horizon of death.*

The specificity of the work of the palliative care team was explicitly named by them in terms that were different from the ones I have just used. At a meeting of members of the two clinics, the palliative care group sought to clarify their areas of concern. They said that they "deal with pain, anxiety, constipation, spiritual stuff and End of Life Option Act." The series, which is hardly a set, is clearly heterogeneous. It would be a mistake to attempt to make a distinction between the two clinics' concerns at the level of the "object" of attention, as though some elements of the illness experience concern the "person" while others do not. What is crucial is that with respect to any given concern, or a specific symptom that requires attention, there are ways of taking up that symptom or concern in ways that either do or do not foreground questions of identity or of personhood, to use some terms that are yet to be given specific senses.

With respect to the ALS clinic, I endeavored to show, concerning communication between professionals, patients, and their families, that while it did serve as a functional means for exchanging information, the ethical stakes of the communication, for the professionals, in my reading, was precisely to manage what could possibly be the excessive demand of making "the whole person" visible by way of englobing evaluations of the state of the patient in the clinic. The ALS clinic operated in a manner that I was surprised by and which could be conceptualized, in the wake of the description in the last chapter, through a distinction, although never thematized, between the patient qua *body-subject-to-illness* and the patient qua *person.*

Anthropologically speaking, the contrast, the distinction, goes against a grain, one that is well depicted by Marilyn Strathern in a broad-brush characterization of personhood in "present times," within medical environments:

> In present times communication is valued for its own sake because it *acknowledges* the patient *apart from* the ailments. Patients may *regard themselves* as a repository of knowledge (they *tell* the doctor things) and one who gives knowledge also should receive it, treated not just humanely but also intelligently. *Here* the whole person makes its appearance as an agent. In short, a rather specific act, sharing information, summons something much more comprehensive—respect for the person as a subject rather than as an object—and that respect in turn (as far as Euro-Americans are concerned) activates the whole person.[2] (emphasis added)

With respect to the palliative care clinic, I would like to ask what, or where, Strathern's "here" indexes. Although my contrast between two interconnected clinics, as well as the endeavor to index the specificity of the ALS clinic, tries to show that the specific "value" of communication (recognition of the person apart from their ailments), of which Strathern writes, is not broadly normative, even within this one particular institutional domain—namely, a given medical center in Northern California with specialist services for ALS—nevertheless, in relation to those specialists to whom questions of how to connect living with illness to the horizon of death are delegated, there is an indetermination and a preoccupation about personhood to which the clinic endeavors to respond. It is in that sense that I think Strathern's concerns about the conditions under which "persons" are made visible and sayable, and the conditions under which they are "hearable," are concerns that are central to the palliative care clinic.

The question, then, is the following: in what way is the one who is subject to a specific kind of motion toward a horizon of death made to appear, within the clinical apparatus, and in what guise? In what way does the subject of the discussion, the patient who has this illness, exist within the palliative care apparatus, for the palliative care workers, and how is the position of this "one who is subject to" oriented with respect to the dual topics of identity and the horizon of death—how is this position and orientation worked on and through by these clinical workers, by way of the technical support of this clinic?

I insist on the specificity of the question: how does the one who is subject of and to the discussion, within the apparatus, appear in relation to the horizon of death for the palliative care clinical worker? The question of the individual's relation to themselves in relation to this horizon will be dealt with separately, in part 3 of this book.

From One Clinic to Another

At the end of August, it was suggested that I sit in on a consultation with Mrs. Liu and her daughter Yu, which was to take place by way of "telemedicine" (using Zoom). Mrs. Liu had been diagnosed five months previously at the end of March 2019. During chart review in the morning, we heard that her illness was advancing rapidly, that she was having a terrible time breathing, that she would like to talk to the respiratory therapists, that her daughter gives her enemas because her bowel has stopped moving, and that she has previously discussed the End of Life Option Act. She is a Mandarin speaker and her daughter translates for her. She had seen the team once already in person but was now too exhausted to make the 50-mile trip from her home to the clinic.

Mrs. Liu began her visit with the respiratory team. They went through the technical issues with the two machines she is using, the Trilogy machine at night and the BiPAP machine during the day. Colette told Yu that she has an exercise that she'd like her to explain to her mother: one deep breath in and then to count out loud. Wei Liu counted in English, got to ten, and then started to say numbers at random. It was roughly twenty. They discussed settings on the machines again. "Is she in late stage?" Yu asked, with respect to her mother's last respiratory results. She was told that sometimes shortness of breath is not reflective of the percentage of forced vital capacity (FVC). In June, it was 40 percent. Colette said that she would not say that Mrs. Liu is in late stage.

"She wants to do it again, to challenge herself," Yu said, referring to the test.

Colette repeated the rules of the game and said that she can do it in Chinese and to speak slowly. She got to twenty again, "Pretty good. Tell her that speaking in short sentences can help if she's short of breath."

The team members passed through the little office with Wei Liu and Yu on the screen, profession by profession. After respiratory it was the dietician, then speech and language, then physical and occupational therapy. Other than breathing, two major issues were raised: frequent urination in the night, which posed a problem with respect to getting her in and out of bed, as well as pain in her lower back, likely caused by spending all day sitting in her wheelchair. Yu then asked if they could see the doctor.

Dr. Blumen came in and said straight away that it is important to get Mrs. Liu's symptoms under control. She suggested directly that she should have a telehealth visit with the palliative care team because they are very good with addressing symptoms related to shortness of breath.

Let me underscore that this way of announcing a passage and referral from the ALS clinic to the palliative care clinic, in my experience, was typical; an ALS clinic physician often suggests the referral. The nuance pertains to what has been said and seen such that the physician makes the referral. In this case, there are two elements: the expression by Mrs. Liu of a demand to make use of the End of Life Option Act during a previous clinic visit, as well as the presence of symptoms that are best attended to, in the view of the ALS physician, by a palliative care clinic.

What is also important to bear in mind here is that with respect to her symptoms, and in particular Mrs. Liu's breathing difficulties, while Dr. Blumen's concerns can be heard as simply a matter of physical symptom management, the palliative care clinic, as we will see later in the chapter, considers themselves adept at addressing aspects of respiratory symptoms that go beyond the technical expertise of the respiratory team at the ALS clinic, broadly speaking the aspects of shortness of breath and respiratory difficulties linked to anxiety and panic. Although she lets the two statements sit side by side without making any link between them, Dr. Blumen then said that palliative care is also the group that Mrs. Liu can talk to about the End of Life Option Act. They are the ones that "prescribe the medicines," Dr. Blumen specified. Wei Liu had not, it should be noted, mentioned medical aid in dying during this visit, although her chart review indicated that she had brought it up previously.

In response to Dr. Blumen's proposal to contact the palliative care clinic, Mrs. Liu spoke at length in Mandarin, which her daughter then translated as, "She prefers experimental stem cell therapy." Yu then asked whether the palliative care team "prescribe medicine," which Dr. Blumen confirmed, specifying that it would concern "medication to help with shortness of breath." Dr. Blumen said that she wished she could get Mrs. Liu into a stem cell therapy protocol, "but now it's about slowing down the rate of weakness, not about reversing the weakness."

"I saw some people on TV walk after they had stem cell therapy," Yu said, interpreting for her mother.

"I don't think they had ALS."

"Do you have any patients on BrainStorm [a stem cell clinical trial]?"[3]

"Yes."

"How are they doing?"

"We don't know who is on placebo."

"Did symptoms slow down?"

"Not obviously. But preliminary data did indicate slowing down of the disease."

"I'm just waiting to die, it's a bitter life."

"First step is to control symptoms. Using the machine more [BiPAP] during the day should make you more comfortable."

"I don't have energy to talk. Are there any other experimental therapies?"

"No. I wish there was something in the pipeline."

"She says, can you and the other doctors urge the FDA [Food and Drug Administration] to accelerate it?"

"There is still a year to go."

"What about Right to Try?"

"The company said yes at first and then no. 'Right to try' means you can approach the company to ask them whether you can try the drug."

"We tried to contact them, but no reply."

"Until proven, they are reluctant, perhaps because so many treatments have made patients worse."

"She sees the TV advertising, sees the people walking again, and hopes to be the same case. Very anxiety [producing]. She is very depressed."

"It's wrong, this false advertising. The thing about 'Right to try' is that it was always the case, and always the case that it was up to the companies to decide."

Yu then raised a question about the two drugs her mother is taking, Radicava and riluzole: Yu wished to know whether her mother should continue using them even though her condition is declining so rapidly. The advice she received was that if there are no side effects, she should continue; if she has side effects, she should stop to see if she feels better. Yu said that she thought Radicava caused her mother's falls the previous month. Dr. Blumen specified that even if she stops Radicava, she can keep in the Radicava port; there is no need to have it removed.

"Before she could raise her arms. Now she cannot."

"Yeah, so maybe now is the time to stop, to see."

"So for stems cells, the only one is in Korea, right?"

"I've had people do that."

"Better?"

"It's not clear if it works."

"Does it mimic the clinical trial BrainStorm?" Yu is asking whether the Korean stem cell clinic uses the same protocol as the one used for NurOwn, by BrainStorm Cell Therapeutics, at that time in phase III trials in the United States.

"Yes, similar protocol."

"Can you get her in BrainStorm? She will pay."

"Well, they had said patients could pay $100,000 and that we'll give it to you, but then they went back on that."

"Can you, with other physicians, push to get them to agree to that?"

"I tried. They refused to do it until the study is over. It's a problem with manufacture, they can't produce enough, they're not being mean. They already had to halt the trial once due to manufacture."

"It would have been better in March [when she was diagnosed]. She feels like she is going to die if you don't help her."

"Everyone in BrainStorm dies too: we don't have anything to stop the disease."

"For the palliative care treatment, do you have to be in the hospital or at home?"

"It's usually very peaceful, go to sleep and then don't wake up."

At this point, it is worth pausing to note that Yu spoke of an indeterminate "palliative care treatment," to which Dr. Blumen's response was polyvalent and could be heard as indexing both the general way in which people die through hospice care, as well as the act of medical aid in dying, something that Mrs. Liu had expressed interest in pursuing previously but who at this meeting had explicitly sidelined this option in order to pursue "active treatment." A second point worth noting is that whereas at the end of the previous chapter, Dr. Blumen had actively blocked a patient from seeking medical aid in dying because breathing scores were too high, here, with the same scores (roughly 40 percent of predicted forced vital capacity), medical aid in dying is actively supported as an option. The element that would appear to make the difference is the apparent rapidity of the decline of Mrs. Liu in comparison to Si Chang's slower decline, which indicated, in Dr. Blumen's view, approximately a year left for her to live.

Dr. Blumen finished the meeting by saying that she was sorry that the disease had progressed so quickly for Mrs. Liu. They planned on seeing her again in a month.

"She wants to be a white mouse." Yu said that her mother was repeating "stem cell treatment" and "white mouse" [guinea pig]. "Why does she progress so fast?"

"Everyone is different, we don't know why."

Making a Person Present

Unlike the ALS clinic, palliative care consultations happen as a single group of multiple professionals meeting the patient, usually with a family member. There is a nurse, a social worker, usually a chaplain, and the physician. As a way of giving a sense of how the clinic works, the kinds of questions it addresses, and the way in which a person appears in relation to having this illness, within the confines of the meeting, I will put into series three instances of clinic visits. To make the obvious point explicit, already in the mere manner of how work is organized and in the very form of the interaction, the fact that multiple medical staff members meet together with the patient (and usually someone who comes with them) means that points of view stemming from multiple professional concerns cross each other during the discussions, thus creating a focal point in and through which the individual comes into focus in a particular way.

Rather than having one point of view follow separately another point of view such that different functional and experiential issues with functions/parts of the ill body can be talked about, one by one (as in the ALS clinic), instead, here in the palliative care clinic, there is a shared orientation to how the patient is doing, a search to specify and answer the question of how those present can make an encompassing evaluation of the state of the person, in relation to the illness, an evaluation that is shared to the degree that this question of "how" is talked about together.

We can see this quite simply in the first instance, in which I sat in on a consultation with Dawn and her husband Dave.

Dawn wore a neck brace, helping to keep her chin up, to stop it from dropping. Sylvie, the nurse, a driving force of the palliative care clinic, brought Dawn and her husband into the room. On this occasion, we were five in the room: the fifth person was a physician, Dr. Sandy, who was finishing a palliative care fellowship.

Sylvie asked Dawn how she is doing and gave a guess to her own question: "crappy?"

Dawn nodded. She had her writing board in her hands. Dawn could not speak. "IT IS WHAT IT IS," appeared on her writing board. An initial refusal of the interpretive and evaluative work that she had been invited to engage in, a begging of the question that presupposes a self-evidence of the situation.

"That's Dawn!" Sylvie said, "that's her motto."

"STILL LOTS OF PROBLEMS GETTING A GOOD NIGHT SLEEP."

"Anxiety," her husband said.

Dawn made a motion with her hand, a downward spiral.

"Do you think you are having anxiety because you can't sleep, or you can't sleep because you are having anxiety?" the doctor said.

"Or something else?" Sylvie added.

"FLEM."

They discussed the BiPAP machine, whether she felt tired in the mornings, and her breathing difficulties, which Dawn indicated stemmed from her chin dropping. They talked about the use of her expectorant, for the issue with phlegm, and discussed whether she was administering the expectorant drug through her feeding tube.

"No tearful spells?" the doctor asked.

"WHEN IM ANXIOUS."

"I SOMETIMES FEEL LIKE CRYING."

"BUT HOLD BACK."

"WORRIED ABOUT GETTING PUGGED UP."

Dr. Sandy said that ALS can cause "mood swings," and she said that the last time they had discussed Dawn's fluctuations in mood, she had mentioned the drug Nuedexta (a combination of dextromethorphan and low-dose quinidine). What is important to note, which was not discussed, is that Nuedexta is prescribed for the symptom of pseudobulbar affect, uncontrolled laughter or crying, a condition in which the person experiences emotions in a normal way but expresses them in an excessive way. Hence, as explored in detail in chapter 2, it is a nuanced point as to whether pseudobulbar affect can be designated as a mood disorder. In any event, when they last spoke of it, Dawn and Dave said it was too expensive—it costs roughly $1,200 a month.

Dr. Sandy asked Dawn whether she would consider something else, another medication to help with her mood. The choice she was given was either mirtazapine (Remeron), which is good for depression but would not treat anxiety, or a selective serotonin reuptake inhibitor (a class of antidepressant).

"ID LIKE SOMETHING TO HELP ME RELAX MORE."

"How have you been?" Dr. Sandy asked Dave.

"Fine." He shook his head.

"How are you doing?" Dr. Sandy asked Dawn.

The doubling of the question to Dave and Dawn opened a space in which precisely a set of crossed gazes will make Dawn appear within the discussion in such a way that an explicit normative question of *how she is doing* is talked about, shared, and worked on.

"I think she is doing amazingly well, considering. She's inspiring me," Dave said.

Dawn then shook her head. Each affirmation of doing fine, or doing well, was accompanied by a shake of the head, for husband and wife. Dave ruffled his own "fine" and Dawn ruffled his evaluation of how she is doing.

"Are you being hard on yourself Dawn?" Sylvie asked.

Dawn began to cry.

The question Sylvie posed followed Dawn disrupting her husband's evaluation of how she was doing. This question produced a signal without words, tears. Dr. Sandy then said that we were in a safe space, Sylvie went to get some tissues, and after a little while during which no one said anything, finally Sylvie turned to a question, which appears technical and somewhat of a non sequitur but in fact had an effect of indexing a question of the horizon of death:

"Is the suction helping?"

Dave sounded relieved by this question to the degree that he jumped in straight away to give an enthusiastic response: "Thank God for those machines! There were a couple of times where she would have died if we didn't have them." Dave's statement opened onto a discussion of how to control saliva, manage constipation, and get Dawn's weight up, and then the question of what she spends her days doing: dog shows and a James Bond marathon on Sunday; she reads a lot, Dave told us; she does big puzzles, she's still doing the bills, she was a ceramist but had to give that up, and she has started doing paintings.

The meeting finished with Dr. Sandy asking Dawn to bring in photos of her paintings the next time. Dr. Sandy summed things up by saying that it sounds as though there are lots of good days, with some challenges. They agree to talk again about goals of care in four weeks: Dawn left with a prescription of Zoloft for the anxiety and morphine for the shortness of breath.

My aim in presenting this first instance is simply to establish how the form of the meeting is capable of orienting how a person can be made to appear within the conversation through an effort to give a broad evaluation of "how they are doing." On the one hand, it certainly is the case that palliative care has "personhood" and person-centered care as one of its ideals and its aims, part of its normative background through which there is a broad orientation that their role is to aid the person to establish their goals of care and for those goals to be tied to a "whole-person" approach, to connect decisions made to a person's wishes and to what is most important to them, in relation to the illness. On the other hand, these goals and ideals have to be put into practice, and as we saw in the last chapter, simply bringing up the issue of identity is not sufficient for questions about it to have an effect.

The efficacy of the question as to whether Dawn was being hard on Dawn, effective to the degree that it produced a sign that was left uninterpreted and led to the issue of revising goals of care, was produced precisely by way of a question from the physician as to how each individual was doing, which opened a space for Dave to say something about his wife, to say something about "who she was for him" (an inspiration, he said), which she then negated, and which then opened up onto Sylvie's question as to how Dawn appeared to herself.

Variations on the Technical Support of the Clinic

Palliative care clinic by way of the crossing of gazes, by multiplying the positions and the possibilities of speech in the clinical situation, makes "a person," as *one* instantiation of the individual-that-is-subject-to-illness, present, to the degree that the individual is invited to say something about how they are. This invitation is a crucial aspect for the normative work of the clinic. I will now contrast two instances of explicit normative work in which the clinical workers make evaluations and endeavor to get the patient and their family to make normative evaluations of their situation. The instances are contrastive simply to the degree that they show opposite combinations of physical and psychological states: in the first instance, the person is not doing badly per se, in terms of motor neuron degeneration, but is suffering severely psychologically; the second instance is then the opposite of the first (significant physical degeneration that appears to be borne well by those concerned). What I wish to present in the instances is how the teams engage in normative work that links *how* the patients are with respect to their illness to *who* they are with respect to their illness.

Sylvie is in the consulting room with Dr. Carly. They had seen Bethany at the beginning of September, six weeks previously. Her daughter Mary had brought her in after an ALS clinic referral. Bethany had stopped walking. It wasn't that she was no longer able to walk; it was that she had "decided" to stop walking. She was catatonic, Dr. Carly said. She had never seen anything like it, except when she was a student and spent several months in psychiatry as part of her rotations. Bethany had been prescribed mirtazapine (Remeron) and methylphenidate (Ritalin). The visit was by videoconference. Sylvie and Dr. Carly sat next to each other, and I could see myself just behind them, and so positioned my head between them in the image of ourselves that we were facing.

Bethany and her daughter Mary then appeared on the screen. Dr. Carly introduced everyone, and then asked Bethany how she was doing. She was doing a bit better than the last time and mumbled, when pressed, that she was sleeping a bit better and eating a little more.

Dr. Carly asked whether Bethany was feeling any more hopeful. She said that she supposed so and that she didn't take the Ritalin, because she didn't want to take that drug.

Sylvie said that this was okay, that their role is just to make recommendations and that Bethany doesn't have to do anything she doesn't want to do. "It'll take some time for the Remeron to work," she said.

Bethany's daughter explained to us that her mother is still in the wheelchair but is able to stand in the shower. Mary said that she was hopeful that the medications would work and that they could help her mother with her concerns about falling.

From the limited amount of information available, it seemed as though Bethany's symptom, her "refusal" or "inability" to walk, was connected to a concern about falling.

Audre, the palliative care social worker, all of a sudden burst into the room, waving, two thumbs up, a bundle of joyous energy. "Uh oh!!! Looks like we're getting a bit of smile!!!" she said, looking and waving into the screen. Audre sat down, and Dr. Carly continued.

"So it was the beginning of September that you stopped walking. Your fear of falling is legitimate. What do you think about home physical therapy and occupational therapy coming to see you?"

Bethany replied that she doesn't have money for that. Sylvie explained that Medicare covers eight to ten sessions.

They discussed how the home visits would work. Bethany told us that she did not think she'd be eligible because her Social Security account had been hacked. Her daughter returned to the concern that the longer she goes without walking, the harder it will be to walk in the future.

Audre asked Bethany to share her thoughts, and she shook her head. Sylvie asked Mary if there are things she's worried about.

"I hate talking about things because I don't want to hurt her feelings, but I feel she has given up," Mary said. "That's wrong for me to say because she really believes it, it's not a choice, but I have a sense that she's choosing to give up."

"This is a difficult illness, the way you feel is a normal reaction," Audre said, redirecting the conversation to Bethany. "But our hope is that we can wedge our way into your inner working, we hope that you can find a few sparks of joy when there is a good day, to see that life is worth living today."

Dr. Carly emphasized that it is important to bear in mind that "it is the depression making the decision not to be able to walk," not "Bethany"; she emphasized that there might well be incremental changes. Bethany's daughter agreed. "Bethany, is there anything that you are hoping for, or looking forward to?" the doctor asked.

"No," Bethany said.

"We talked before about things you used to like to do. Maybe those are some things that Ma [mother] can be on the lookout for, if there are moments when you might like to do some of those things?" Dr. Carly asked.

"I talk about that all the time" Mary said.

"Families are the most important things for us," Audre said. "Growing up, I am sure that Mom insisted on doing certain things because there were things that it was important to do, now the shoe is on the other foot. There is a deep connection between you two. Bethany, I'm trying to speak to you, these recommendations are being made because we think they can help you, none of them will harm you. I see those birds in the background [behind Bethany and Mary, on the wall]. What is that, are they ducks? Those ducks, flying. And at some point today, I want you to look behind you and see those soaring birds, those ducks, and to take a step in the direction of flight!"

"Shall we check again in three weeks?" Dr. Carly said.

Beth mumbled.

"Mom doesn't want to, but I do."

They agreed to a follow-up appointment, and we said goodbye.

Dr. Carly asked her colleagues whether Bethany had a referral to the Memory Center, which is a specialist clinic for diagnosing frontotemporal dementia and atypical dementias. Sylvie said she did not think that it is really worth their time. That she was referred from ALS to the palliative care clinic in March (over six months previously).

"She must have been able to speak enough then to be able to decline a visit from palliative care," Dr. Carly said.

Audre summed up the situation. "The trouble is we have elements missing: we don't know about her history, we only have the daughter's view; she says she wasn't like this before. I think the daughter is right, that she is hopeless. . . . Identity loss is so extreme for our ALS patients."

"It's there in all of our patients," Sylvie said, "but it's an extreme end of the spectrum."

"Did she ask for EOLOA [End of Life Option Act]?" Audre asked.

"I wouldn't prescribe for her if she did," Dr. Carly said.

"Right, but is she suicidal?" Audre asked.

Dr. Carly said that they had asked about that the last time. "She's so apathetic she's incapable of doing anything. Her daughter is there all the time."

"Right, but the risk is if she starts to feel a bit better. . . ." Audre didn't finish her sentence. It was time for another appointment.

I would like to present a last instance, a discussion with Richard and his wife Sandrine, to give a contrastive case to that of Bethany, one that is contrastive to the degree that while physically, Richard is in a seriously limited and perilous state, psychologically he says he is doing very well. In the scene, it is less the case that the patient is *made* to appear as a person; since everything was said to be going "great," there was no work to unpack further how he was doing. Rather, we see how the team makes an evaluation of the decision, a year previously, to undergo tracheostomy and invasive mechanical ventilation, making his breathing dependent on a machine, an evaluation that turns on the family support structure that he benefits from, linking how he is to who he is, considered an effect of the social link that supports him.

The team asked Richard how things are going. He had been in the hospital. Richard speaks through a text-to-speech device activated by ocular movement. His replies to questions posed to him are not elaborate because of the time and difficulty in typing by way of eye movement. Sylvie began by saying they were aware that he had been in hospital and then asked him how things were going overall. He replied that that they were "good." Carly asked what in particular was going well, and at this point, Sandrine gave a more detailed reply. Richard went into the hospital to get a new feeding tube put it. It had gotten clogged three times: "The first two times we managed to unclog it ourselves, the third time we went to the hospital, and they weren't able to unclog it so he had to have the tube replaced."

"Everything is going good," Richard added.

"It got clogged because the food was too thick, we tried diluting it, but that didn't work, so we had to replace the tube."

"Who's helping out at home with you?" Audre asked.

"My eldest daughter moved out, but she helps. We're just off the waiting list for a night nurse. I've been the 24/7 carer for the last year. If I need to go to the store, my son or daughter comes over. So in terms of carers, there's me, my daughter, and the night nurse."

"That's a great addition, hopefully allows you to get some rest at night."

"I sleep when he sleeps. Sleeping is okay now. Everyone helps out, my ten-year-old is in elementary school and she even knows how to do the suction."

Sylvie explains to us that Richard also has a son who took over Richard's bakery. Sandrine tells us that the bakery is doing well.

"What else has been on your minds?" Dr. Carly asked.

Sandrine told us that Richard is typing. Meanwhile, Sylvie whispered to me that he is "full code," meaning that if his heart or breathing were to stop, any medical professional attending to him would do everything in their power to keep him alive.

"Nothing much," Richard said.

"Anything uncomfortable? Shortness of breath? Anything bothersome?" the doctor asked.

"No," Sandrine replied.

"You're feeling good in your body now that you have your feeding tube replaced?"

Richard said yes.

"Anything challenging for you all?"

"No problem," Richard said.

"I'm really impressed," Dr. Carly said.

Sandrine told us that she always calls two weeks ahead for his medication, in case they have a problem: "I have two calendars, one for who is coming to the house, and at what time, and the other one with the medical appointments."

"Wow, that's impressive," Sylvie exclaimed. "What did you do for work?"

"Before I met Richard, I was twenty-three years in child care."

"I wanted to check in how your spirits are?"

Sandrine said that Richard liked to make fun of people. "We go to cheerleading practice three a week and the games on Saturday."

"Amazing," the team says in unison.

"I got a van, Richard is my front passenger so I can keep an eye on him, then I just need a new suction machine."

"I know you met with Sylvie and Dr. Timothy when you were making the decision around tracheostomy and ventilation: is there anything we can be helpful with?" Dr. Carly asked.

"We're having a party on December 6th to celebrate one year of trache and feeding tube . . . they told us normally people die after six months."

"I can hear the joy about how things have gone unexpectedly well," Dr. Carly said.

"They gave us a time frame and we got past it . . . so I just need to think of a new milestone."

"Yes, day by day . . . very inspiring."

"We're going to go back to the farmer's markets to see his friends."

"Remarkable job, not only extra time but quality time."

"When he got trache/vent, he wanted to get out, to communicate, he didn't want to be stuck in a room."

"You've done a remarkable job making that a reality. . . . And we want you to know that we're also here when things change, or if there are symptoms preventing you from doing what you want to do."

"When the cheerleading season winds down, we'll visit funeral homes to get things in order; I don't want to have to rush like with my daughter, who I had to bury in a rush. I hope he's like this for another four to five years . . . but it's also good to be . . ."

Richard intervened: "We proved the surgeons wrong."

"GREAT JOB!" Audre shouted.

"They are happy to be proved wrong," Sylvie said.

"Ha ha ha" Richard said.

After the end of the visit, the doctor commented that Richard is one of the few people for whom tracheostomy and mechanical ventilation "is a reasonable decision." What Dr. Carly did not say is that Richard is one of the few patients to have made the decision in advance about how he wished to see the illness through into its last stages, which for him meant living as long as possible with the aid of mechanical ventilation.

Orientation

Richard and Bethany were polar instances of how individuals are able to work through bodily changes, and the instances combine to show different ways that the palliative care team endeavors to assist patients in adapting to bodily changes, as people. The significance of the next instance stems from the fact that it is a first meeting for Jack, who has ALS, and his wife Linda, with palliative care. The specificity of the instance is that is shows the couples' and perhaps especially Linda's concern to get oriented toward a horizon of change, as well as to get Jack to face that horizon.

"We've read a little about you, but notes don't always reflect your experience. Now before asking how you are, maybe I should give a little bit of our spiel, to let you know who we are and what we do." Linda pointed out to the team that she actually requested the appointment, and in a gesture that was tricky to place, somewhere between gracious and ironic, she told Dr. Carly to go ahead anyway with her spiel.

Dr. Carly explained that a big part of what the team does is symptom management: "maximize quality of life, advanced care planning, and then make sure care matches what you want. Okay?" Jack said yes. His wife commented that he is a man of one-word answers. She then explained why she requested the visit: she has been a health care professional all her working life, recently at a major hospital in administration, and now works in research, "and I've been through this with family members."

"What do you mean by that?" Dr. Carly asked.

"Going on two years, I lost my sister to scleroderma."

"So more experienced than you'd like to be."

"Than anyone would like to be. And I'm a planner."

"What work did you do, Jack?"

"Union carpenter."

He worked massive projects. It was hard work. Audre noticed that they live in a small community known throughout Northern California for its charm. They have been there twenty years, Linda said to the team.

"I think it's going to be good going through this now, to be with a community; very strong community."

"Sounds like the sort of place where everyone knows everything."

"Yeah, for better or worse . . . we actually run a dog rescue and the dogs are good therapy. The dogs know, they stay very close to him, they know when I'm upset."

A discussion ensues about which ALS clinic they are being seen by and what physical therapy Jack is doing. The ALS physician had cautioned him to limit activity, but Linda said that they are people who like to keep moving, she thinks he should get the right kind of exercise, and it would be good if there were something they could do together. Margaret the social worker called the day before and they "talked needs": they talked about speech and language issues, about doing speech banking and recording set phrases, as well as a word bank, for down the line.

"At the beginning overwhelming, last night talked more, he's willing to do it now, that is maybe our next task."

"Yeah, record my one-word answers."

Dr. Carly said that she had been able to look at the survey they had filled out prior to the meeting and that "breathing" and "the future" were listed as Jack's main concerns. When prompted to say more, Jack said that he was worried about losing the use of his hands, about being wheelchair bound and about not being to talk. He specifies that at that moment, it was more "inconvenience" than anything else. Audre echoed that they are legitimate concerns.

"One thing I will say, Jack, in my work with ALS patients, it's very common, you're used to your body cooperating, and suddenly for it not to do so, that's scary, it's worrying. One thing I've been really surprised by is how if those things should change, people find ways of adapting, and still find significance, whatever that may be. . . . If I can ask, in your life, have there been moments where you have had to adapt?"

"Yes and no: I'm pretty stubborn at times. My wife can verify . . . I'm worried about her having to take care of me."

"This [illness] is unexpected . . . but if the shoe were on the other foot, I'm sure you'd want to take care of her; it's important to recognize how hard it is to receive this [care], when we're used to giving, it's hard to receive . . . we're here for you all. We might not be able to stop you needing a wheelchair but we're here for you."

Dr. Carly then brought up that she saw in the notes from neurology that Jack is not taking either of the possible medications sometimes prescribed for ALS. She asked why not.

"Should I say something?" Linda intervened. "That conversation with Dr. White at ALS Clinic was a little contentious, he brought it up, I work in clinical research, so I'd researched the drugs, one is not very good, and the other extends life span two months, are you kidding? Drugs reach markets because there is nothing else. He put in the notes, 'The wife declined the drugs,' he even put that in the notes! He suggested the drugs now, which I think is premature. Plus, we do alternative medicine, acupuncture, he didn't even want to put it in his notes. Jack has osteoarthritis, overlooked during diagnosis and confused the diagnosis; I had requested an MRI of the upper neck and back. With construction work it's a very common condition: a doctor at a different hospital helped sort that out, acupuncture helps with pain; numbness in hands attributed to hands, but in fact carpel tunnel, due to hammer hand. Now diet, common herbs mitigate spasms, magnesium. It's not that I'm against drugs, I work in the pharma industry but I see the whole picture, one of the things in the plan going forward, that we look at those options; I call it a dual track."

"You won't find dispute in our team: we'll help you define what you want in your care and help you orchestrate that. We have seen very little progress with people on this medication: risks and benefits; I'm really glad that you're educated about it, have looked at both sides of the page, and made a judgment. If acupuncture works, great! Our job is to figure out how to support you."

Jack then proffered that he takes Zoloft and another medication for his prostate. "I was diagnosed with what they call depression. I didn't think of it as depression. I was angry, at myself. Lashed out at my wife, I have memory problems and sometimes I forgot."

Linda told us that "this journey to ALS" has been almost four years: going on four years, she noticed mood changes and what she called lack of follow-through on tasks. "I work for a company that works on statins, family has history of cholesterol, in the rule-out process, to figure out mental issues, he didn't think he was depressed, but the physician thought it was but then the ability to concentrate got worse, then I mentioned speech and motor issues."

Audre then said that it is her duty to inquire as to whether he ever has suicidal thoughts. "The last time the psychologist asked, I said why do I have to pay my bill first! I never thought I was depressed; the drugs help me with what I'm going through, I see some of my friends going through the same thing and they don't think of themselves as depressed." Jack talked a little more about other areas of concern, such as breathing, and he did not answer Audre's question.

"Were there other things you were hoping to talk about?"

"Well, for way down the line, what end-of-life services are available?"

"Do you have things in mind?"

"No, I want to know my options."

"Have you drafted advanced directives?"

Linda said that yes, they had, but that they need to discuss those, because it says no feeding tube. Audre reminded us that these documents are "fluid" and that a feeding tube "maybe is a valid choice."

Mrs. Liu, September 2019

Most people do not make a decision in advance about how they wish to live the final stages of ALS. Nevertheless, since 2017 in California, there has been one more option to consider in advance, for that minority of people, in addition to tracheostomy and mechanical ventilation—namely, "medical aid in dying." In the remainder of this chapter, I will return to the story of Wei Liu and her daughter Yu in order to narrate a particular set of events in which several of the elements that I have named so far appear as indeterminations to be considered. The first essential and basic question, in relation to Mrs. Liu's rapidly accelerating illness, concerns what she wants; what does she want to do in relation to how she is living the illness, with respect to what appeared to be a rapidly declining state of her body? A response to this question was complicated by the question, stemming from Yu and her mother, of what the palliative care clinic could offer and help with. From what I had understood from the meeting at the ALS clinic, Mrs. Liu wanted to know how close to the end of life she was and to use that information to make a judgment about what could be done in relation to that end. The starkly contrasting options, at least the first time I sat in on a clinical consultation with her, were her apparent request for information about "medical aid in dying" and her insistence on wishing to be a "white mouse," to have access to an experimental stem cell treatment that she hoped could cure her.

In a very small consulting room a few floors down from the ALS clinic, one month after the first time I met Mrs. Liu and Yu, Dr. Sandy, Sylvie, and I sat getting ready to meet with them over a video link. Dr. Sandy had read through the ALS clinic notes and was aware that I had sat in on Mrs. Liu's last visit with ALS clinic.

"So you've met her already and she wants to talk about EOLOA?" she said to me.

"When we met, she didn't mention EOLOA," I said. "She did talk about stem cell clinical trials, about the FDA, and being willing to pay any price for a possible treatment."

"Oh boy," Dr. Sandy groaned. "Okay, well, I bet it comes up in the last ten minutes and we're gonna get sucked into at the end. We usually wait for the patients to bring it up."

Sylvie was irritated because they had put in a request for a translator who had not showed up. She went to see what she could do about it. I mentioned that at the last visit, there was a translator there, but quickly it became apparent that Yu was translating very efficiently, and the translator quickly ceded his role to Mrs. Liu's daughter, saying that she was very good.

The video interface started to ring. We all introduced ourselves. Mrs. Liu was in her wheelchair with her BiPAP machine. Yu was sitting to her right. Confirming my impression from the previous ALS clinic visit, I was struck by Yu's straightforwardness. To the question, "How are you?" Yu gave a synthetic account of the situation in which they were living: "There is a caregiver at night; I don't work in order to look after her in the day. My mom says she is not feeling well, she has difficulty breathing, she cannot move, all four limbs are too weak to move. Prior to June, she was able to walk. Then in June she began to fall." Mrs. Liu says something. Yu laughs, something I had noticed at the last visit, a nuanced message, or sign, certainly not making light or making fun of a situation that she acknowledges is distressing, but perhaps an alternative to tears, an expression, a sign linked to the affective investment in communication with a health care team for which there was at least a hope that something could be done to ameliorate her mother's situation.

Or, perhaps her mother had simply said something funny.

". . . yeah, she says she is disappointed about the BrainStorm phase III clinical trial. We expected the results at the end of 2020, now delayed until 2021. I cannot wait to see the results; I will not be here to see them. She says I wish the FDA would approve it, but they don't let me try it. She says thinking of these things makes me hopeful. I [Mrs. Liu] wrote letters to the FDA and BrainStorm, but they don't answer."

"Yes, regulations are very tight," Dr. Sandy said.

"Phase II already showed safety, why two hundred patients need to be enrolled in phase III with restricted eligibility? She says, I don't want a cure, just something to improve quality of life, I tried riluzole and Radicava, but stopped both because of side effects."

Dr. Sandy apologized for having gotten a little ahead of herself in asking how Mrs. Liu was doing before explaining what the palliative care clinic does.

Yu carries on with the previous discussion, "And she says, if you have opportunity to talk to the FDA to expedite the process." Sylvie, who is not on screen, sitting in a chair next to the computer, says to the rest of us in the room, but not to Mrs. Liu and Yu, that no they do not have a direct channel to the FDA.

Dr. Sandy confirms what Sylvie said, saying to Yu and Mrs. Liu that they don't have a channel to the FDA.

"Okay, but it's hard. How can you help?" Yu asked.

"So let me explain what palliative care does," Dr. Sandy said, whose tone and manner had shifted to an expository mood. "We take care of people with serious illness. We can help with three aspects: we are the experts in helping people improve their quality of life; then we want to know what is important to you, what good quality of life means to you; what your values are; we want to make sure that treatments given are in line with your values. Then lastly, we also help with supporting the family and caregivers of sick patients."

Dr. Sandy followed up by saying that she heard that Mrs. Liu was hoping to get into the clinical trial in order to get better quality of life.

Mrs. Liu spoke. "Yeah yeah," Yu said, "She says, I want to participate, even if I have to sell everything I have."

"What is good quality of life for you?" Dr. Sandy asked.

"At last I can take care for myself, to not be dependent, no shortness of breath, easy to breathe. Maybe some independence," Yu said for her mother. "She just goes in her wheelchair every day, in the wheelchair in the morning, then back into bed at night."

"Why doesn't she go out?" Sylvie asked.

"There are three reasons," Yu said, quick as a whistle, "One: Breathing machine is huge, so big it's hard to bring it out. Second reason, even with the electric wheelchair, which she moves with her fingers, eventually finger gets tired. Third reason, bathroom, not convenient if we go outside."

Sylvie then asked how many hours of BiPAP she does a day.

"Twenty hours. And the symptoms are getting worse."

"So really big changes," Sylvie said, making a simple overarching evaluation of the situation.

"So, once the fall on the back of her head, then symptoms come on quicker."

"I am so sorry, I can see that this really," Dr. Sandy pauses for a moment, to find the right word, "sucks. When someone starts to get breathing problems like you have, there are medications to help with breathlessness."

"What do you mean?" Yu asked. "Less frequent BiPAP?"

"No, less feeling of shortness of breath."

Sylvie, who is still sitting facing us, in line with the computer, hence out of view and out of earshot, said to Dr. Sandy that the morphine can be used in combination with the BiPAP; they are not exclusive.

Yu clarifies that "using the BiPAP is still okay, it's when she isn't using it that she feels breathless."

"So you can keep the medication at home just in case. Also, if you feel breathless, try opening the window to feel air on your face."

"Dependence?" Yu asked, referring to the morphine.

"It's a tiny dose," Dr. Sandy said.

"People react differently," Sylvie then specified, leaning over to talk directly to Mrs. Liu and Yu, "sometimes people can feel drowsy. If that happens, you can decrease the amount."

"Can the medication protect her breathing from getting weaker?"

"It only treats the symptoms, won't prevent muscles getting weaker," Sylvie shouted, from her position off-screen.

"Even taking medication, she needs the breathing machine, right?"

Yu, in my view, was endeavoring to parse what exactly palliative medicine does, whether the medications and interventions proposed were aimed at reversing the symptoms (which they are not), hence grasping what is meant by a medicine that is palliative rather than curative. Through the discussion, Yu understood that what is being suggested is a low-morphine dose to help with breathlessness, so that her mother can go outside a little bit without having to take the BiPAP machine with her. Mrs. Liu seemed pleased about this, Yu told us, to be able to go outside.

Dr. Sandy suggested trying the morphine at home first, to see if it helps and then, if it does, to try going outside but not too far. She suggested going to the porch first.

Sylvie wrote E O L O A on a piece of paper and showed it to Dr. Sandy, who then transitioned delicately to the topic: "On your survey, the number one thing you said that was a problem was feeling dependent on other people. Tell me more about that."

"My mom says I [Yu] don't go to work, and that she is a burden she is worried about her daughter, I [Mrs. Liu] always disrupt normal life, and there is no way to treat this disease."

Sylvie intervened, leaning over to the screen: "Yeah but if your daughter was sick, I bet you'd want to help her no matter what."

"Yes, because I'm her mother," Yu said, "she's young, it's different. She has children to raise." Yu has a one-year-old at home. Sylvie said that she "accepts" that Mrs. Liu "does not buy" her argument.

"You're living together?"

"Yes."

"That's nice."

"She cannot accept that this disease does not have any treatment. It's completely unacceptable to her. Dr. Blumen said prognosis of one to six months, what does that mean?"

"It means at the current stage of disease progression, most patients live another one to six months."

"She says so I have no chance to wait for a trial or therapy, probably in one to six months I will die."

All of a sudden there is lots of loud talking between Yu and her mother.

"Did she just say assisted dying?" Sylvie asked.

"Do you have this service?" Yu asked.

"Yes."

Dr. Sandy intervened, "We hear this a lot from older ALS patients, being a burden on their families."

"I'm not old, I'm getting worse, too much suffering."

"I hear what you are saying. We will need to talk about physician-assisted dying."

"Right now we cannot discuss?"

"I can give you an overview, but I don't want you to rush."

"Okay, yes, give me the overview."

"Basically what happens in the process is that we will need you to give us two voluntary requests fifteen days apart. Then a written request, in general we can do that on the second meeting. Then we need two physicians to confirm that life expectancy is less than six months."

"Dr. Blumen will be that physician?"

"We would be the clinic that prescribes and Dr. Blumen would be the physician that confirms the prognosis. Based on this meeting, less than six months, it's always difficult to say, but I think yes, I worry that we may be at that stage."

"I wish we had her breathing numbers, I think they were in the fifties last time, for us we'd need them to be in the thirties," Sylvie said.

"So it's mostly decided by breathing? If she wears the machine every day, how long before respiratory failure?" Yu said.

"It's very unpredictable," Dr. Sandy replied.

Yu then asked whether even with use of the breathing machines, if respiratory failure could happen at any time.

Sylvie replied clearly, "Yes."

"I'm afraid, yes," Dr. Sandy confirmed. "All this is very difficult news to hear. Let me just finish going through the steps. In the fifteen-day period between the two requests, you will talk to Audre, who is the social worker."

"So today is the first mention?"

"Yes."

"So what happens after fifteen days, we can cancel, right?"

Sylvie intervened, "The medication stays in the pharmacy. If you never want to take it, that's okay. You can always change your mind."

"During this period, I will still hope that the Americans come up with a treatment."

"We hope with you," Dr. Sandy said.

"The most important part," Sylvie underscored, "is that you have to be able to do it yourself, to drink the medication."

"She cannot lift her hand," Yu said.

"Can she drink through a straw?" Dr. Sandy asked.

"Yes."

"Someone can hold a cup and she can do it, is that okay?" Dr. Sandy asked, although it was left unspecified in what sense she meant "okay" and to whom exactly she was addressing her question. Two senses of "okay" are evident: first, physically for Mrs. Liu to do the act and, second, legally for someone to intervene in such a way to make it possible for Mrs. Liu to end her own life, in accordance with the law. Sylvie made a face indicating discomfort, which I read as linked to the second point.

"Yu, are you okay with this?" Sylvie asked.

"Not sure, I don't want her to suffer. How does it happen?"

"Once she takes the medicine, she will fall asleep and won't feel anything in a few minutes."

"It usually takes how long to die?"

"Four to six hours, sometimes a lot less."

"No pain, no breathing problems?"

"The medicine takes care of breathing problems and no pain."

"If no pain, that's good."

Sylvie specified that it is not covered by insurance and costs six hundred dollars.

Mrs. Liu, November 2019

After a second meeting in which Mrs. Liu and Yu talked about the possibility of going to Korea, they met again with the team for a third time. Sylvie tells us that Mrs. Liu has just come out of the emergency room (ER). She had been short of breath and "choked," with Sylvie adding the quotation marks with her fingers, and had to go to the ER. Now Mrs. Liu says she wants EOLOA. "Man, that's not how we do it. We want you to plan!"

"It makes me uncomfortable," Audre said.

Sylvie tells us that Mrs. Liu doesn't want to go back to the hospital; she wants the meds at home. Sylvie would like to revisit the benzodiazepine and the opioids. The team discusses whether removing BiPAP use could be an alternative to EOLOA, but that may only work if she were taking benzodiazepines. Hence, it could only work if she were willing to try that again.

The team is ill at ease at the prospect of approving medical aid in dying for Mrs. Liu. As a way of marking this malaise, it is noteworthy to contrast her request with that of another patient, Mr. Jerri, who made the request at roughly the same time.

Mr. Jerri is in his eighties and lives in rural Northern California in the middle of a national forest, roughly 400 kilometers from the palliative care clinic and a long drive to the nearest hospice, medical facility, or other amenities. He met with the full palliative care team, including the chaplain, three weeks earlier by Zoom. That he made a new "telehealth" appointment in order to talk about medical aid in dying was confusing for the chaplain, Dr. Zara Lange, because he hadn't brought it up the last time they spoke. Sylvie told us he called back right after that last appointment to arrange this discussion, saying the she thought he didn't want to say anything in front the friends who were with him during the visit.

Mr. Jerri told the team that his symptoms had started to move up to his arms. It's progressing faster than he thought. "I'm looking down the road," he told us. The team asked him whether the Radicava has helped. Both he and his family who were with him on the consultation said it's difficult to know, since there is no point of comparison. It's going quickly, and there is no hospice in the area. Mr. Jerri asked practically how it would work. The team told him that a pharmacy would FedEx a prepared set of medications, along with instructions. They require two days' notice and it costs six hundred dollars.

The chaplain interrupted the practical discussion to ask what "death with dignity" meant to Mr. Jerri. "I don't want to suffer," he said. She asked him whether there were things he wants to do before he dies. "Things I gotta do," Mr. Jerri said, matter of factly, "sell a piece of property, move some money around." The chaplain reiterated her question, asking if in terms of relationships there was anything he wanted to do.

"What?" Mr. Jerri did not catch her drift.

Mr. Jerri's daughter-in-law translated, "Anything you wanna say to the boys?"

"They just lost their mother [died of a stroke]. I think they'll understand, they won't want me to suffer."

"Have you got particular thoughts about who you'd like to be there?" Dr. Lange said.

"No. No one needs to be there."

"Be nice to give them the option, though," Mr. Jerri's daughter-in-law said.

"Yeah. I'm definitely sure I want to do this."

Mr. Jerri's request was received by the team as not requiring any probing. Audre the social worker was able to do the "psychiatric evaluation," which is not a legal requirement but rather a hospital policy. She ensured that he was not being coerced. His was a case of an "independent person," as the team described him, a man in his eighties who lives in a rural setting and hence would have limited access to facilities if he were to live longer with the illness, a "straight talker" who does not want to suffer. His request appears as, on its own terms, self-evident.

By contrast, Mrs. Liu's request, her changing attitude, the lack of control over her breathlessness, and her and her daughter's vacillating plans including, inter alia, going to Korea, solicited concern from the team. At this critical meeting, the third with palliative care, one of the more senior palliative care physicians is present, Dr. Clara. Sylvie suggested that in addition to the EOLOA discussion, perhaps a psychiatric evaluation from outside palliative care should be requested. In saying this, Sylvie knows that she is increasing both the time of the procedure and the risk of a refusal, since an independent psychiatric evaluation would be more stringent. Sylvie, Audre, and Dr. Clara discuss what they worry to be a lack of reflection behind the request and begin to raise concerns about Yu's role as translator. Sylvie goes out of the room to try to find a translator but comes back alone.

The meeting starts with the question of what happened when Mrs. Liu went to the ER. Yu explains that her mother took a dose of lorazepam (barbiturate) at night before going to bed; she then had increased nasal secretions, and in the morning, when Yu measured her mother's heartrate, it was at one hundred. Dr. Clara assures Yu and Mrs. Liu that the heartrate was not due to the lorazepam. Dr. Clara asks Yu what her mother was doing such that she took a dose of lorazepam; she took a shower. Yu asked what could have made her heartrate go up, to which Dr. Clara replied, "Lots of things can: worry, anxiety certainly can, and the lorazepam might be a useful tool for that."

"She says if she continues to get worse, she will take the end-of-life option."

"Would you be willing to try the lorazepam again?"

"No. She is saying no."

A discussion ensues as to whether she would be able to be off the mask for longer if she were willing to try the benzodiazepine again, as currently she can manage only a few minutes. Dr. Clara thinks this is unlikely but that the medication could help her feel more comfortable while on the machine.

Dr. Clara then gets to the heart of the matter: "There is something we really want to understand: you made the request to have medication to be able to end your life: what is making you request that?"

Yu laughs and says, "I just told you: given my condition and no effective treatment."

Unfazed, Dr. Clara says, "There's a lot of truth to what you said: it's not a life that everyone wants to live. Our team is just making sure that it is a consistent wish, that you are feeling confident and consistent in your wish, not just today."

"You are right, she is saying she wants to do that, it's not something she can change, it's a decision she makes with the progression of the disease."

"Yu, is this a consistent wish?"

"Yes. She's saying, can you prescribe the medication sooner, wants to go to hospice and then take it there. She doesn't want to die at home."

Dr. Clara tries to clarify what soon means. Yu says her mother is concerned about suffocating, that the visit to the ER was painful, and that she wants to see how things go over the next weeks. Everyone agrees that the plan is to see how stable she is over the next few weeks, how tolerable the situation is, and for Mrs. Liu to see what she can adjust to.

Audre picked up on a crucial detail. "One important thing that we need to share," she said, "is that we don't know of a facility that allows people to take it [medical aid in dying medication] in their premises. You would have to take it at home." Audre then asks whether Mrs. Liu has a hospice service, which she does, and given this second request for medical aid in dying, regardless of whether Mrs. Liu ultimately takes the medication, the team suggests that Mrs. Liu should be switched to hospice care, meaning that no new life-extending measures should be taken.

Audre asks how Yu feels about the plan: "Maybe it is good for her, after the visit to the hospital, the tube down her throat, it was painful, the tube made her voice difficult, I feel this decision is good for her and good for me." Yu comes back to her mother's wish not to take the medical aid in dying medication at home. Sylvie asks if there is not a facility that would allow her to do it on their premises, whether she would take it at home; Yu says no, that she would look for another location. "She doesn't want to do it at home."

"One of the recommendations is not to do it in a public place," Sylvie said.

"And how is it for your husband, Mrs. Liu, is he aware?"

"He respects her decision."

"One last thing, we need to make sure that this is her independent wish."

"How will you ask her?"

"Can you tell her to nod her head if this is her wish, or to shake her head if it is not her wish, and then you go away from the screen."

Mrs. Liu nods.

"That's a big nod!"

"Can I come back?"

"Yes."

"She was very clear."

Mrs. Liu, December 2019

Audre was about to call Mrs. Liu and Yu on Zoom. "I'm not going to do a full psychiatric evaluation with the screen, because of the language barrier. I'm most interested in the fact that it is very rare for a Chinese or Asian family to make this choice, so I'd like her to talk a bit about that." I asked Audre what else she took from the last meeting. "The main thing was at the end, she said she didn't want to do it at home, that she wanted to go to a facility to do it. Well that's going to be a problem."

"Hello Mrs. Liu, hello Yu. It's good to see you. I'm Audre, the social worker; this is Anthony, a visiting researcher from France, whom you met last time. I'd like to continue the conversation about having asked for End of Life Option." Mrs. Liu nodded. "Can you tell me more about how you learned about it?"

"We asked about this to Dr. Blumen, who referred us to your clinic."

"You are Chinese; it is rare in my experience for Chinese, or Asians, to do this. Can you tell me a bit more about your decision-making?"

Mrs. Liu speaks and then Yu translates. "I don't want to be a burden to my family. I don't want to wait because there are no effective treatments. I learned about it already when I was healthy, from books and media."

"I think you are incredibly brave: many people say they value it [medical aid in dying], but not as a real choice."

"I make this decision because there are no effective treatments."

"It is heartbreaking. You worry about being a burden: what else do you worry about?"

"She is worried about getting worse and worse."

"That's a real worry, to not have control about how your body will change. Some people have ideas about what happens to their body as they get closer to dying. Do you have any ideas about that?"

Ms. Liu shook her head and then spoke. "I thought about the disease spreading but I didn't think about my body at death."

"Some people are worried about things like shortness of breath, pain, losing their dignity, are any of these a worry to you?"

"She thinks about shortness of breath. Worried at that point will suffocate."

"That's why we have you monitored with palliative care."

Yu didn't say anything to her mother. "Translate that please," Audre requested.

"Two medications prescribed, but neither work."

"How did you feel when they didn't work? Emotionally how did you deal with that?"

"I'm upset."

"Did you get so upset that you cried? Did you feel dark?"

"I'm not depressed and I don't cry, because then I can't breathe properly."

"That's rotten! That's not fair."

"Yes, she feels that it is not fair, why is this happening to me? What I do to have this? On the other hand, I'm still concerned for my family and grandchildren." Audre asks Mrs. Liu to say more. "Family back in western China. I was hoping there would be a miracle."

"Yes, you have to balance hope, being in the present, and the reality of your body changing."

"She was hoping a breakthrough would happen soon, so the patients could be saved from the disease."

"We're still far from that: given that, what does bring you joy, or engage you with your family? How do you spend your day?"

"They are busy taking care of me, and of the children. Now I just want to get this started so it is ready."

"I want to go over logistics, but before I do, let me ask, if you didn't have this option, what would you be thinking about?"

"No, I never thought about it."

"I want to make sure that since your diagnosis, you didn't think about taking your own life because you are so sad."

"This medication won't hurt me: no pain."

"Sometimes people have ideas about being ready to take it; what will be the conditions when you say: I am ready to take this medication?"

"If the disease continues to progress, I will take the medication."

"During the last couple of weeks, she stabilized; once she reached the point of being on the mask all night, she stabilized."

"I know being on a mask is hard, but you seem to have adjusted well."

"Not comfortable, but it's the only option."

"A necessity, even though you don't like it."

"Another concern: she doesn't want to do it at home."

"I am concerned about that: What are you looking for?"

"Facility."

"The law says it has to be in the home setting. So that is one of the issues."

"Can it be out of California?"

"No, this law is specific to California. I need to understand why you don't want to be at home?"

"Worried that if she does it at home, it will become a bad thing to the whole family."

"A bad spirit, a bad omen to the family?"

"Yes."

"My worry," Audre said, "is that once we prescribe the medication, it is part of her medical record. No facility can have a nurse or doctor help with it. The medication must be mixed by the patient or a family member."

"Okay. She understands."

"What is she asking?" Audre requests clarification from Yu as to what her mother is saying.

"What does it mean on medical history?"

"A prescription on her record, just like all other medical prescriptions. The law in California allows providers to participate or not."

"I can mix the powder at the facility."

"Who would be the person you would ideally like to be the one who mixes the medication?"

"My family, my daughter."

"You would want your daughter. I would want you to understand what it would mean for you, Yu."

"Initially I feel like I am killing her. But I feel it is the only option we have."

"It is hard to realize you are following her wishes. But it is not an easy thing for you. Does it make you sad, or uncertain?"

"Sad. If I am following her wishes, then maybe I will feel better."

"Your intention is to be of help, to be of service."

"She is helping me."

"It's important for the two of you to talk between the two of you."

"She feels uncomfortable in this position," Yu said, referring to her mother's back pain.

"We'll need to talk again. Let me say this: I don't see undue influence, no reason to not let you do it, but I will need to talk to you again to make sure you understand how the process works."

"Next time we talk about process."

"That's right. Bye bye."

Emergency

The events that followed this conversation were not totally unexpected, although the exact turn of events was not predicted. After the psychological evaluation at the beginning of December, Ms. Liu and Yu refused a follow-up appointment request to talk about the "process," as Audre had put it. At this point, no prescription had been established for the medical aid in dying medication. Important to recall is that once the prescription is made, it is sent to a collaborating pharmacy from which the patient may request the medication at any time. The pharmacy then sends the lethal medication and instructions to the patient, who then manages these themselves, although frequently in dialogue with a home hospice or home nursing worker, since being able to request the medication goes in tandem with being "on" hospice.

On December 30, 2019, Yu called palliative care, and a prescription was established. Her state was declining. On the night between January 1 and 2, she was taken to the emergency room, and the patient was confronted with a choice between dying and having a tracheotomy and then going on invasive mechanical ventilation.

Mrs. Liu chose the ventilator.

Part 3
ONE BY ONE

Part 3 changes the way in which ALS is able to appear as an object of attention, as well as the way this object of attention is taken up: away from medical knowledge and clinical care practices per se and toward the question of how those who have ALS work on living with it; work here signifies using language, writing, and speech to work on and through the manner in which they have a body with ALS and how they have knowledge of the illness while having knowledge of their singular experience with this illness. This question (of knowing and having) is one of orientation: a question regarding those things that individuals living with ALS are oriented toward and one of how they are oriented toward those things, a question of disposition—indeed, of relative disposition—given a form in language.

In the second part of the book, the work of the clinicians, in the ALS clinic, was explored, and that work, I claimed, was oriented by a kind of functional grid that bracketed questions of identity: an initial column indicating the individual, noted by way of their initials, analyzed by way of a sequence of functions, along with the exponent of the matrix, the doctor function. In a palliative care clinic, the coordinates were provided by explicit normative work on the question of "the person," rendered explicit through crossed gazes, and within discussion, between those present at a given consultation, about *who the person is*, for those present at the encounter in the clinic and how those present in the clinical encounter view the person with respect to the horizon of what is to come. Part 2 thus endeavored to provide a response to the question of how clinical practitioners countenanced the ones who presented themselves in the clinic with this illness. I described countenances within the institution, in these two different clinical settings, broadly indicating two orientations, which should be understood in terms of how they differ. The one in the ALS clinic explicitly bracketed personhood and questions of identity, in order to separate knowledge of body functions from a question of any possible sense or meaning that could be given to knowledge of that body, knowledge that, for the most part, concerns degeneration of body functions. This orientation, and this countenance, I argued, was not a consequence of normative negligence, or indifference, but is actually itself a form of normative work. The other attitude, in the palliative care clinic, was observed to have then unbracketed the question of personhood, a setting in which clinical practice confronts the patient and those who come with the patient to clinic, with the concern as to who the person is, in relation to knowledge of this illness, degeneration, and the time that remains.

What is at stake in part 3, then, is the "medium specificity" of language, harnessed and invented by singular beings who have this illness, in which and through which individuals orient themselves through coordinates beyond the clinical, beyond those of body functions, and other than that of personhood.

Part 3 is thus composed uniquely of three narratives, in which I ask, one by one, how three women have oriented themselves, in having ALS and to having ALS, and what (else) they have been oriented by while having ALS. The narratives are told chronologically: the first is about Frances, being a written account from the 1970s; the second and third narratives are about Emma and Gwen, beginning in January 2020, with Emma's coming to a close when she died and Gwen's an open-ended narrative, breaking off as she continues her work and her search for treatments. I tell the stories chronologically rather than thematically and singularly, rather than all together, because although there is something universal about this illness, being universally fatal for those that have it, that universality does not encompass how its current incurability is worked on and through for each person and what becomes possible for each to work on.

What I take up in each of the three narratives that follows is how points of signification can be identified, the medium in and through which they are identified, and how they function as coordinates—points of signification, in which and through which, and relative to which, singular human beings living with ALS tie themselves to or else endeavor to grasp themselves within an experience of ALS—I put it this way so as not to say "point of view," a phrase that can be misleading, if taken literally, as well as if taken as a metaphor. I wish to avoid the presumptive orientation that the anthropologist could somehow grasp an "experience," per se, the phenomenological *Erlebnis*, of the one who lives with, the one who is thrown into a situation of having, this illness.

The three chapters that follow explore my preoccupation with the idea that my wanting-to-know about life with this illness has something to do with not only "the person" but also, to put it more accurately, what this particular illness makes sayable and visible for and about the one subject to this illness. While the narratives that follow show how specifically cruel the illness can be, they also reveal the sometimes surprising ways in which people work with and through situations and the invented mediums through which they put their subjectivity to work, which does not therefore mean that they necessarily adapt to, or reconcile themselves with, the situation.

I focus here on three ways that three individuals use mediums through which they work on how they are oriented to having ALS. These three mediums are the "epistle," the "plea," and "advocacy." While far from being exhaustive, as a series, they provide variants with respect to the parameter of address. Who—in which position—is addressed by whom, and in the name of, or toward, what?

Very simply, the epistle as a written medium concerns an object of attention, with questions and reflections written from the "land of ALS," as Frances Mc-Gill puts it, addressed to an audience, who live in an elsewhere, and with didactic intent by an individual, McGill, writing from the position of an inhabitant of that other place.

The plea differs to the degree that it is a form of demand, and it is addressed to (one or) another (person), and rather than being a didactic undertaking, it is, at base, a request for love. I take up the story of Emma, whom I met three months before her death and not long after she had her medical-aid-in-dying request accepted, a demand that opened out onto the indeterminate concern of "when" the right time would be to do it. Her concern with timing was connected to her own claim that she was supposed to "learn something" from her experience, a something that was intimately tied to a working through of her personal history and her relationship with God. Her plea is vitally connected to her search to know something about God's love for her.

Lastly, what I have called the medium of "advocacy" is enacted again by an individual, Gwen Petersen, but in her case as *one* of a collective, a patient-led activist nonprofit organization, called I AM ALS, participation through which provides orientation toward, search for, and re-search in hope of repair, considered in its multiple significations, a search for which she has made it her work to advocate.

I have given just one variable or parameter through which to consider this trio as variants, namely, from whom and to whom an address is addressed and the medium of that address. This is a first indication, then, that medium here indicates the specific modes and forms through which an individual endeavors to be heard or read. Following Rosalind Krauss, the specificity of each medium must be sought in the support and the materiality of the medium: in the case of Frances McGill, the epistle as medium is supported through the use of writing, the letter as form and as signs, in Morse code, a specificity of the medium that is integral to her practice within the epistolary medium. With Emma, the medium of a demand for death must be grasped within a spiritual practice connected to knowledge of God's love. For Gwen, the medium of a search for hope, in research, is supported by a collective mobilization for more urgent action and in the "call toward" (the root meaning of the term *ad-vocacy*) action.

Very simply, medium as a question of "who" is the subject of or in speech, or writing, cannot be enclosed in the referent of the illness: it is for this reason that the "illness experience" is the last thing the anthropologist could claim to grasp, to the degree that it is impossible to grasp, being graspable only to the degree that words are extrinsic to any supposedly transparent referential meaning. As an example of that impossibility, it suffices to recall the person in the last chapter, Dawn, whose tautology "it is what it is" gave those present the sense that they both knew what she was saying and that it stood in for who she was—"that's Dawn," the nurse replied—because, of course, in a certain sense, Dawn is absolutely right; it is what it is. And yet, we have reason to wonder whether Sylvie, the nurse, is right in the same way; it is what it is, but then what could it mean for that to "be Dawn"? Indeed, the point of the last chapter was to underscore how an englobing image of the person is produced, which the nurse achieved absolutely. That is the power of that particular clinic. And yet what is at stake here, at the end of this book, is thus precisely to ask, at the point at which speech crosses with language, how the subject who speaks about their experience of illness through speech and writing introduces a gap and an opening, in relation to what could be indexed as a point of contact with the real that this illness brings into existence, as well as how to live with it, and despite it.

EPISTLES TO ONES

A set of letters, close to two hundred pages, by Frances McGill, written from "the land of Amyotrophic Lateral Sclerosis,"[1] between 1974 and 1980, the year she died, although published before she died, began, very simply, not as an account of, or else a narrative about, illness, nor as an autobiographical undertaking, nor as a project to document living with this illness, which these letters also, in part, can be read for, and come in part to provide, as they go on; rather, initially, they were a means of telling her "Dear People" and her "Dear Ones" that their loving messages and gifts, sent following news of her diagnosis, had given her a "warm wonderful feeling": "how are you to know," she stated plainly in her first letter dated July 18, written from home in Roxbury, Massachusetts, "unless I tell you?"

As bulbar-onset ALS symptoms began to show, as Frances McGill was forced to give up her job as a community worker in the Boston neighborhood that had by the 1970s become the center of Black culture in the city, as African Americans from the South moved north from the 1940s and 1950s onward, as her speech became slurred, and as she lost her "beautiful singing voice," in the words of her childhood friend who also grew up in Turkey with her, both of them as the children of American Christian medical missionaries, she began to write, "producing two volumes of memoirs and semifictional sketches of her exotic childhood".[2] Frances McGill knew what genre of work she was engaged in, when it came to writing something about living in relation to an experience of illness—epistles.

It is precisely the work that a letter does, what she was engaged in, as well as the laboriousness of the process of writing letters that she will come to submit to, which is of concern for me. The epistolary genre was a choice. Soon after she began to write these letters, however, she became deprived of the physical capacity to speak. The letter as a form remains a choice; nevertheless, it was a choice of how to make use of a sequence of particular modes of communication, physically produced one single letter at a time, modes that she had recourse to once she lost the capacity to speak, modes of communication that came to be her only means of exchange, once her physical capacities diminished to the point at which she was able to move only her eyes.

The book of letters can be broadly divided into two parts, corresponding to two phases: a two-year period from July 1974 to July 1976, during which she lived at home and could use her hands to write or type, even once her capacity to speak was gone, and a three-year phase after July 1976, up until June 1979, during which time she resided at the Jewish Memorial Hospital, in Roxbury, a situation that would remain unchanged for the remainder of her life and which is the period that accounts for the large majority of her letters.

Early on in this second phase, during which she was "utterly unable to speak" and unable to move her body, her friend from church, Mary Mae Tanimoto, suggested that she use Morse code to both communicate her needs as well as to write. She could indicate the code by right and left movements of her eyes. She was then subsequently able to make some use of a machine then in development from the Tufts University bioengineering department, the "Tufts Interactive Communicator" (TIC), "which responds through a delicate switch to very slight movements of her head and generates a ribbon of typescript."[3] Lastly, when the technical aspects of the machine became too difficult or even impossible to manage, for McGill and those whose assistance she required, she made recourse to a "simple board" that showed the letters of the alphabet, such that even someone not versed in Morse could read her messages.

We have seen in prior chapters some devices and techniques patients use to communicate when they can no longer speak. Again, it is McGill's practice of writing that concerns me, not the quasi-vital operations of communication. Nevertheless, her reflections on this quasi-vital aspect of communication, in her writings, are precisely of interest to me. McGill more than once reflects on the vital importance of those around her being able to decipher what it is she wishes to communicate to them. The concern for communication is hence both linked to, and also distinct from, writing letters as a medium whose purposes will require consideration and which I think can be qualified as a way of working with, and through, this experience of illness. It is precisely because of the particularity of this work that she undertook in these letters sent from McGill to the group of "Ones," "People," "Dear People," and the "Dear Ones," a mode of address that I will endeavor to show enables a reader to partake in that address, to receive what is written in the letters as something to be considered.

The specificity of the epistle as form distinguishes consideration of McGill's work from an analysis of the autobiographical genre, into which most first-person writing by patients with ALS can be put. Recent examples include the interactionist sociologist Albert B. Robillard's *Meaning of a Disability* (1999), the writer Frédéric Badré's *La Grande Santé* (2015), and the historian Tony Judt's *The Memory Chalet* (2011), to name just a few of those intellectuals who lived and died with ALS and sought to give form to their experience in writing.

My concern, as a reader of McGill's letters, is to ask what letter writing, as opposed to memoir, autobiographical narrative, or the essay form, provides in terms of medium through which to work on, if not through, an experience of ALS. In setting up this concern, I am trying to be clear about my starting point, that while it is undoubtedly the case that "writing" is a general term for the use of written language as a medium, and it is a practice that people have recourse to in order to work over experience, nevertheless it is also a term that is a little underspecified. We are dealing here with letters. And if the question "what is a letter" is perhaps slightly too academic, one might wonder nevertheless how, in terms of material, form, register, and address, the letters take on functions as letters, as well as the purposes to which letter writing is put, which is to ask, what do these letters do? Peter Sloterdijk's reply to Martin Heidegger's *Letter on Humanism*, "Rules for the Human Zoo,"[4] which begins by citing the Romantic poet Jean Paul (Johann Paul Friedrich Richter, 1763–1825) to the effect that "books are thick letters to friends" and that letters are "telecommunication in the medium of print to underwrite friendship," although a little one sided, and hence ideal-typical, nevertheless has the benefit of well-identifying that one side, which is to say, the aspect of demand within a letter, a demand for love, in this case, *philia*.[5] A demand for recognition is certainly how McGill's letters begin.

Beyond demand, if McGill is supposed to learn something through the work of letter writing, however, it is not of a didactic nature; indeed, the letter seems to occupy a crux point between the bodily experience reflected on and any possible or impossible search for understanding drawn from that experience. A question I will endeavor to answer is to what extent the work undertaken in these letters, even if not properly speaking didactic, can be characterized, nevertheless, as "working through" (*perlaboration* in French; *durcharbeiten* in German), in a relatively strict psychoanalytic sense, a sense given definition in Rycroft's critical dictionary: "Working through: Originally, the process by which a patient in analysis discovers piecemeal over an extended period of time the full implications of some interpretation or insight. Hence, by extension, the process of *getting used to* a new state of affairs or of *getting over* a loss or painful experience. In this extended sense, mourning is an example of working through, since it involved the piecemeal recognition that the lost object is no longer available."[6] It is my contention that there is analytic work on the place of loss within subjectivity going in these letters, and it is also my contention that with respect to "a new state of affairs," the question that is precisely open, opened by the work of these letters, is what "getting used to" or "getting over" could possibly, or impossibly, signify for a subject, what kind of reorientation it involves, work that is positioned between knowledge of an experience, and the bodily changes created by illness.

Communication

Go Not Gently: Letters from a Patient with Amyotrophic Lateral Sclerosis begins with a letter from physician Arthur E. Reider to McGill's father, Albert W. Dewey, also a physician. Important to note is that Reider was a psychotherapeutically inclined psychiatrist. After studies at Harvard, he conducted an internship at Mount Zion hospital in San Francisco in 1965, which had become a major center for the development of hospital-based psychoanalytic treatment in the Department of Psychiatry, established in the 1930s by European émigré analyst-physicians Dr. Bernard Kaufman Sr., Dr. Ernst Wolff, and Dr. Leona M. Bayer, among others, and headed for many years by Reider's father, Norman Reider, chief of psychiatry and senior psychiatrist at Mount Zion. After revealing Frances's diagnosis to her father, "almost certainly bulbar onset ALS,"[7] Reider explains that he is seeing her once a week. We can infer that McGill continued to see him up until her hospitalization and even after she lost the capacity to be understood by way of speech, devising instead a practice by which she wrote letters to him, and he then read them aloud, in her presence, and talked about them with her.

She explained to her friends and family that she had decided to send them some of these letters that she had written to Dr. Reider, concerning her work with him, because she thought "it fitting for you to read some of this discussion because it is a continuation, in a way, of the 'dear people' and 'dear ones' epistles."[8]

Again, with this in mind, it is possible to insist on the very simple sense that something other than "communication" is going on in the work of these letters, even if communication is a key topic: "the contents are kind of strong stuff," she warns, "and might give some of you indigestion, in which case don't read it," she advises. "It isn't necessary . . ." she trails off, the ellipsis functioning as her own accentuation of the open question as to what exactly is not necessary. She then clarifies and, it must be said, underscores the perfomatively verbal quality of the letters that, in spite of their form as writing, stand in for her lost voice: "I mean, I'm not trying to drag you though every minute detail of my experience, unless you want to 'come see' with me."[9] A lot turns on what it can signify to "come see" with her, in addition to the effect of having her words, to the letter, be given voice, her voice being her lost object, given voice by another, in her presence: it is not communication, it is not a voicing to share "every minute detail" of her experience, it is an engagement in accompanying her in her work on her experience, such that something becomes "visible," to use her scopic metaphor, and sayable, if we stay with her description of what happens with her psychiatrist and about which she tells the reader little.

Reider explained to McGill's father that he had consulted with her neurologist, her social worker, a physician friend of hers, as well as her son Paul. "So far all her needs are being met," he wrote. "She is able to feed herself small portions of liquid food and able to get about as usual. Welfare medical assistance and disability have been applied for. People are available to shop for her if necessary. Paul knows the diagnosis and hopefully will be talking with someone at Harvard Health Service to help him adjust to the news."[10] McGill's son Paul was at that time a student at Harvard, graduating a year after his mother's diagnosis. "Frances is not overwhelmed with the prospects," Reider continued, "and is going ahead in a realistic and brave, but not overly proud fashion. She is accepting help graciously."[11] She was fifty-three. Reider was, it seems, instrumental in organizing multiprofessional care, *avant la lettre*, coincident with the emergence of a concern to provide this kind of service, which I have already documented.

McGill's first letter comes three months after Reider's, and so roughly seven months after diagnosis. Her starting point or rather points, since they are actually a set of topics that will come to be given an arrangement, are decisive, given what has already been observed in terms of how personhood is bracketed and unbracketed in clinics today. The topics are "personhood," "rights," "speech," and "truth": Who has the right and the obligation to speak and hear the truth? What is the relation between speaking a truth and considering the addressee of speech as a person, or else of being a person who can hear and speak the truth? The topical geometry is variable.

The way in which these topics were named was articulated as follows. "Dear People," July 18, 1974: "Perhaps some of you could join me in a discussion of something I have been thinking of adding to the 'manuscript' pile, viz.: What are the 'civil rights' of the terminally ill? A good deal has been written in an effort to study and understand something that is mostly surrounded by such emotional repercussions for many, and by folk-custom and by just plain superstition that finally a 'dying' person is not permitted to be a person at all but becomes a sort of property of the 'living' who begin to then work out their own needs with reference to whatever their concepts are of what dying means, regardless of the ongoing 'liveness' of the one with a terminal illness."[12] One of these "rights" that she addresses is the right to know the results of the multiple tests a patient undergoes in the process of trying to reach a diagnosis, not least that of the electromyogram. McGill says of herself that she was "unjustifiably trusting" that she would be told the results of the "painful tests" to which she was subjected to reach a diagnosis and that she was under an erroneous "delusion" that doctors are "mature human beings" who are "more knowledgeable than most with regard to the dynamics of human feeling."[13] Given this error, that she had assumed that she was in relation to someone who would, at least minimally understand, in line with the citation from Strathern earlier, that the one who gives information should also receive it, she was "embarrassed to ask for the results" of her tests, "feeling that such a question was a kind of over-dramatization of the complaints which took me to the hospital in the first place."[14] She continues, "That was four months ago, and I still might be wondering what the hell was happening if it had not been for a different good doctor-friend (outside of Massachusetts General Hospital) who had the consideration for me as a person to call and obtain the facts."[15] This friend was Reider, who took on the role of announcing the diagnosis to both McGill and her father.

Frances McGill writes that she "shudders" for those who are not fortunate enough to have the right contacts. This is then the first way in which personhood, rights, speech, and truth are configured: the patient has the right, should have the right, to be told the truth. Hence, the physician should have an obligation toward the person. This is not self-evident. In August 2019, almost a half-century later, during my orientation to the ALS clinic, a senior neurologist explained to me that the American Academy of Neurology has explicitly named as best practice that the patient should be told once the physician has made a diagnosis, which is to say, it did not go without saying.

McGill gives a somewhat sardonic read on "the young neurologist" who did not tell her the results of her tests and the probable diagnosis. He was trying to spare her, or spare himself, she wrote—sparing himself the trouble of having to be bearer of a lost cause. McGill ironizes, "It is darn inconsiderate of the patient to be terminal and thus cause other people emotional distress."[16] She is frank about the fact that friends avoid her after learning something new about her illness, usually from someone else, underscoring that her "difficulty" with speech "devastates some" because they do not know what to say: "that is, such individuals avoid me since *I* am the unpleasant subject."[17] She is reflective about the fact that her approach to being the unpleasant subject is to develop a "frankness" and "matter-of-factness," which "eases their fright." Their fright of what? From the context in the letter, it is clear McGill thinks she is easing their fright before the phenomenon of dying; nevertheless, there is also room to read that she is easing their fright before the unpleasant subject that she takes herself to be, for them, for herself, which cannot be reduced only to some kind of primary anxiety about (the phenomenon of) death, projected onto others.[18] As a clear indication of just some elements that should be taken into account, in the fore-word to the book of letters, family friend William L. Nute Jr. ended with can-dor: "Frances is terrific, but she's no saint. She can be pretty difficult."[19] Easing their fright could be read as her way of showing those others that her illness is part of her singularity, which included her being "difficult," "matter-of-fact," of not being a "saint," rather than her specificity, as a subject, being reduced to the particular "difficulty" of the illness to which her body is submitted, which would then negate or deny her own singular unsaintliness: "There are people who romanticize illness, and particularly death. That is, they seem to think that sufferings and the prospect of dying transform character, so they expect that a pickle of a character turns into something like jelly, all pliable and saccharine. My dear friend Vicki hints at this kind of thinking when she comments, 'Knowing you is so reassuring . . . the fact that you are dying hasn't changed you a bit. You are just as nasty as ever.' It is true . . . I am not posturing to im-press either heaven or hell."[20] Her curiosity and humor are part of that singu-larity, in addition to what comes across as her being "difficult." She was glad to know, for instance, that the word she had heard used many times in connection with her disease "was spelled 'fascicular' instead of 'vesicular' the latter having made no sense at all to me and the former explaining what the doctor was check-ing when he asked me to open my mouth as wide as I could . . . I felt a little less humiliated by a few episodes of inappropriate crying or laughing when I under-stood the nature of it."[21] A subsequent letter told a story of having gone to a wed-ding where she found herself talking to George Rosenthal, a doctor she used to work with in the Roxbury Community Health Clinic: "And I said something to him which struck me as being really funny . . . I said, 'George, ALS has cured my high blood pressure. This apparently is one unusual effect of ALS. So, if any pa-tients come to you with complaints of high BP, all you have to do to effect a complete cure is to recommend that they go get a wallop of ALS.' George, who enjoys the absurd, began to laugh and then stopped short, looking pained."[22]

At the beginning of September 1974, as speech became increasingly difficult for her, meaning that she had to use paper and pencil when wishing to be un-derstood in public, in shops, for example, she wrote that what she wanted to "talk about is _COMMUNICATION_." She reflects on the typography:

My emphasis on that word via all capital lettering plus underlining may seem disproportionate to its importance at this point of insertion. Like, why not lead up to it gently, subtly, humorously, instead of using a bludgeoning approach? . . . Those of you who are suddenly finding yourselves deluged with volumes of my communications may be wondering why I have to go on at such length, not that you don't like hearing from me, but it becomes somewhat of a task to have to do so much reading. Also, there must be some question as to whether I am expecting equally voluminous responses. So I tell you now that my missives impose no obligations on the recipients of them. . . . In some ways I am simply being a reporter.[23]

These missives, reports that oblige no return, are then the counterpart to the increasing difficulty to be heard, something that McGill clearly wants and that constitutes a loss: "My subject matter will not necessarily interest everybody. Some of you can even develop a sort of form letter which reads, 'I hear you,' and routinely send it off at whatever seems appropriate intervals to keep me happy and feeling that I have been acknowledged."[24] Her suggestion of a standard reply form for "hearing her" is counterpart to the compassion she says she feels for those friends who try to understand her speech through what she calls an extraordinary amount of concentration. Her "slow labored delivery and the long focus on the one portion of my visage," her mouth, which was watched with desperate concentration by these friends, has a "hypnotic or drowsy effect," dazed expressions grow, "or the other person may become so tired that the power to interpret becomes lost so that, for me, the effect is much like talking to a deaf person."[25] She became discouraged from trying to speak spontaneously. It is in writing, she then writes, that she is "relatively free and unencumbered. It is even possible to remain relatively spontaneous via the written word."[26]

Loss

The first mention of mourning appears in her letters in October 1974, six months after her diagnosis. It takes time to confront the loss on which work is to be done. It is in fact relatively uncommon to be able to "hear" from people with ALS because usually there is an initial phase of approximately six to nine months in which a person tries to confront the shock of the diagnosis, getting reoriented to the actuality of the situation, and then, often after that moment, begins a period of decline in which advancing symptoms means that the person is effectively getting ready to die, a period of another six to nine months. Not very many people have time in between, time in that gap, to say something: I think this is what brings together the cases of Frances McGill and Gwen, of whom I will write in the last chapter, and that distinguishes them from Emma, whom we will encounter in the chapter that follows, even though their situations, that of McGill and Gwen, and their historical moments, were very different—bulbar ALS in a woman in her fifties diagnosed in 1974, institutionalized two years later, and a woman in her thirties diagnosed in 2016, who five years on from diagnosis still has the capacity to speak, as well as a degree of mobility and independence. Both Frances and Gwen had time to give form to things they wish to say and to write in relation to living with an experience of ALS, whereas Emma's reflections were very closely parameterized by what she felt to be the impending event of death, and as we will see, her demand to bring that event closer, something that was not present in the same way for either Gwen or Frances.

This is not, however, to say that it was absent in the same way for the latter two. Very schematically, I would say that because of sociohistorical timing, the specific nature of the illness, the singular orientation of the two individuals, McGill was able to engage in a working through of loss, in the strict sense named above, within a medium of writing. Gwen, for her part, confronted her own experience of loss through advocacy work oriented to striving for better access to drugs and medical attention for those diagnosed with ALS, today and for those to come, an orientation to a future on which she seeks to leave a mark.

McGill's first mention of mourning is in the one and only letter included in the book that is addressed from her to Dr. Reider, dated September 22, 1974. It begins with contemplation on her emotional lability, her "stew of tears and laughter," and she tries to both take account of the neurophysiological cause of the excessive bouts of crying and laughing, of which she insists the former are more problematic than the latter, and also focus on what those tears (especially) signify and do for her: "Why my strong alarms and objections to the kind of crying I have done on the occasions of the last 2 visits?"[27] She describes it as a kind of vital weakening, "some basic bulwark or structure is torn away," and a feeling of "crumbling" emerges. This description of a feeling of crumbling and weakening is then worked over with respect to something the pair had previously discussed: during their session a fortnight earlier, Reider was reading her letter and he read aloud the following that McGill had written: "I hope, I do so hope that I am never so unreasonable as to require that you have to point out my unreasonableness to me."[28] McGill "was referring to demands I might make on you [Reider] which were out of proportion to your realities."[29] McGill was concerned about being uncontrolled, affectively, and that this lack of control extended to being excessively demanding, a worry about being "unwittingly difficult"—whereas being wittingly difficult, broadly, seemed to be just fine.

Without the connection between the thoughts being entirely explicit, the concern about being unwittingly demanding is connected to the anticipation of losses to come, which she knows is real, and she wonders about whether or not such *anticipation* of losses to come, mourning those losses to come, is "appropriate" or not: "It occurred to me that despite my disclaimers, I might actually be grieving about losses caused by my death, although I couldn't be sure whether I was then grieving about the loss of you or of me or our relationship, when I got home after that [appointment], . . . I did try to look at that possibility more directly and became aware of deep anxiety and depression that was hard to shake off, get rid of, work my way out of."[30] She became sure, she says, that this work was in fact mourning, in particular "the loss of speech and other growing limitations and disfigurements, which losses in turn cause the loss of certain facets (important ones) of relating to people who are dear to me."[31] The depression she refers to is then qualified as a "continuous process of mourning": death, in her terms "does not occur all at once. I die by degrees."[32]

At the same time, there is a crucial aspect to her experience of loss that is not gradual: McGill insists on the fact that while there are many people who are disabled, unable to use oral communication, in her case, loss of speech was recent and sudden, an event that provides a specific situation in which, on the one hand, at least up until her hospitalization, a part of her, as well as other people, could continue to imagine she had no speech problem at all—for example, she writes of her son Paul asking her questions from another room and wondering why she wasn't answering (much to the annoyance of both)—and, on the other hand, she was terrified of the further losses to come.

What is important to pay attention to is the particular signification of the different losses, ones that she is well aware affect her first and foremost on the narcissistic register of the imaginary: she writes in *A Subjective Report from the Land of ALS (Zone of Frances McGill)*, included in the letters, that "even before it was determined that I had amyotrophic lateral sclerosis, I had to accept that I had a speech defect"—she slurred, she skipped syllables, the speaking voice that she says she unconsciously prided herself on, the voice that "was an important function and projection of me," a device that could sooth and comfort, cheer and inform in her work as a psychiatric nurse and advocate at the Roxbury Comprehensive Community Health Center. She sounded drunk. She did not know it could get worse. "The hoarse quality of my voice and the slurred indistinct speech affected like me like a defacement or ugly scar . . . it was a disfigurement to my psyche, my ego, my self-image."[33] The ugly scar as metaphor, defacement of her countenance, countenance of her defacement.

The diagnosis, confrontation with a cause, was really a relief: "The effort to cope with this disfigurement and continue to work as a psychiatric nurse so exhausted me that I was enormously relieved to be told by the neurologist to rest for a month, and later, by a psychiatrist, that my illness was terminal."[34] Dying, she says, did not disturb her as much as her defacement did. Yet her "habits of self-identification" did not die all at once either: "I form images of myself with respect to how I think of myself in relation to other people. As in the 'squealing baws' I have become a creature who makes distressing moaning and crying noises and one with whom no one can relate, not even me!"[35] McGill makes available the split between her *self* as image and ego, and the *creature* that is subject to these changes; logically, the *subject* is an effect of the existence of this creature whose cries exist relative to language, as well as the loss in the image of self to which she is subject.

Between June 15, 1975, and October 10, 1976, there were no letters. We learn that as of autumn 1976, she was in fact in the hospital and no longer writing her letters herself, dictating them to her "interpreter," a Harvard psychology student named Thomascine Pippin. She called the letter that they were writing their first major project together, and she expected it to take several days. It was her friend from church Mary Mae Tanimoto who had read that the eyes are not supposed to be affected by ALS and who came up with the idea of Morse code, a solution to what McGill called, regarding her incapacity to express herself, her "mute fury."

This first letter from the hospital was addressed to "Dear Cy," one of the members of the Nute family, with whom Frances McGill spent time, growing up in Turkey. She told him that she thought it might be the beginning of another Dear People letter, rather than a Dear Cy letter, and asked him if he would agree to be in charge of a project to copy and send out the Dear People letters to the people who are dear to her. In this letter, located somewhere between Dear Cy and Dear People, she described her first conscious moment on waking in the hospital: "I seemed to be in a dark room that is my remains. You see, I thought I was dead. Some shadow seemed to be creeping along the wall of the corridor. The impression was that they were of two opposing teams: one was friends of Frances. The other team was friends of someone else whose remains were also somewhere in the building."[36] Her next conscious memory was of having been moved to a different room. Her bed was by a window: "It was late at night. The moon was shining round and full. I waited at the moon with sadness for many reasons. I thought about my marriage to Paul's father. I thought of Paul alone without his mother who was dead or dying in a hospital nearby. I cried because I was not dead and still had to die before mourning."[37] Clearly, she did not want the morning, and mourning, to come before she died. It is at precisely this point in her letter work that a word, a signifier, appears in the text: flaking. "The word flaking flashed across my mind in connection with death. It was like reptiles shedding their skins or birds molting and had an aura of oriental mythology. When I was finished flaking, my spirit would soar free in the form of a bird."[38] She came across the word "flaking" in the hospital: a word "for a form of meditation like peeling down the layers of an onion." She says, several months into her hospital stay, after the initial disappointment of not having died, when everyone expected her to die quickly, she slowly came to terms with being alive and to have a "voracious appetite," an appetite that is tightly bound and wound to writing. It was the letters she received from her Dear People, she says, that brought her "to terms with the fact that I am still alive after all these months."[39]

Brought to "terms." Terms is not a synonym for anything that could be called reality. To the contrary, she describes a kind of fantasy work in which flaking produced "a series of composite awakenings": "First, I thought I was surrounded by people in a comedy. Most parts seemed to be taken by friends in disguise; a few unfriendly characters sneaked in. Friends were comically made up. Paul [her son] played every imaginable part and kept appearing, but without seeming to acknowledge me. I reported this fact with grief to someone, as his impossible business deprived me of his company. I also said I found the play very amusing. But I was glad that it was only a play. A voice answered, 'It may be funny, but it is really happening.'"[40] The fantasy also had what she called a "contradiction" that, in addition to being a play, a comedy, she also "imagined that after they arrived, these friends discovered that I was still alive, but most of them didn't come near me."[41] These friends spoke of intimate things that McGill either didn't know about herself or had forgotten. These others, these friends, had taken on the source of knowledge about her. "As these facts became known to my gossiping friends, they became judgmental and took sides for or against me." She says they also seemed angry that she didn't tell them where she was. Of course, she couldn't tell them, but she also became worried midst the comedy that "some ones" were trying to kill members of her family, such that to protect them, she had to conceal even their names from flashing through her mind. In a quite literal reading of the image work happening in this fantasy, we can connect the game of personas, of masks and dressed-up characters, with the narcissistic wound that she is subjected to at the level of her image of her self, her voice, her face, her body. These personas standing in, she says, kept appearing "without seeming to acknowledge her," and thus she could try, only try, to occupy a blind spot in the game of veils. More speculatively, the work of writing, I would like to suggest, was the work she chose to undertake to endeavor to occupy a position as a subject, despite the surprising and novel bodily mediations produced by illness.

Indeed, it is the case that she did not give up endeavoring to form an image of herself, despite her defacement, and in spite of these body changes, which is to say to acknowledge the separation between what was happening to a body, it was of course hers, but to not identify uniquely as that body, to have one without being one. For example, McGill wrote eloquently of the experience of pseudobulbar affect, a passage worth quoting at length:

> One effect of ALS is that certain emotional breaks seem to be ineffectual. I have already experienced some of this, been aware while it was happening that I was not as upset or as sad as my crying would imply, nor as uproariously amused as my uncontrollable laughter would indicate. Such episodes of laughter and tears may have slight connection with my actual frame of mind or the feeling which is actually mine at the time. In fact, I usually become very frustrated and angry at my inability to put a halt to such ridiculous behavior! I begin to smile, but the smile becomes an exaggerated grin, which attaches itself, fixedly, to my face and I have to use all my powers of concentration to remove the embarrassing grimace. If I yield to the impulse, it becomes the onset to equally uncontrollable giggles, which in turn so embarrass me, that I become angry, humiliated, and subject to uncontrollable tears it is a vicious, see-sawing circle! . . . I am mortally afraid of squealing bawls. They destroy me—they weaken and crumble me . . . those deep debilitating agonizing episodes. They are no gentle rain. They are more hurricanes! For me, tears are no longer healing, but laughing is fun if it does not continue so long as to give me an aching solar plexus. You have no idea how terrible it is when the crying is fully triggered and takes hold like a seizure. I can't control any of it. I simply disintegrate and it isn't only emotionally horrible with me, it is physically painful and debilitating.[42]

She wrote these things in a "report" on her experience in the land of ALS, which she had given to "a young neurologist," unnamed in her letters, who came to talk with her, who I have surmised was Aubrey Lieberman, who along with Frank Benson wrote a paper about emotional lability in patients with ALS. After reading her reports, he told her that he wanted to visit her once a week. McGill, now four months into her hospitalization, had begun to wonder what was going to happen to her, since, apparently, she was not going to die, yet she did not know "what was going to become of me . . . I didn't know where I was going to reside."[43] She was concerned about where and how she would stay in this institution. For reasons unexplained, she did not divulge her suspicions or worries; she thought she had to be sly and so tried to get information about where she was going to reside by asking the young neurologist where they would meet. She was too subtle for the young medic, who retorted with the naive optimism of someone who may not yet have heard the words he uttered, "It depends on in which room you are happiest."[44] McGill says that she didn't know when she was "at all" happy. "Happy," she wrote, "is a word which I automatically translate into radiance. When I could write or sing or play the organ or walk a mountain trail or share a beautiful moment with a loved one, I had radiant moments. Now such hours were no longer except in memories. I did look forward to Paul's coming each day. . . . If radiance was impossible, what was valium?"[45]

Valium

Valium is a word, a signifier, McGill began to use in her letters, which in addition to being the trade name for diazepam, a tranquilizer, antispasmodic, anticonvulsant, is "also used here in a symbolic sense to mean T.L.C (tender, loving care), which is often soothing to anxiety-ridden, agitated or otherwise disturbed persons."[46] She attributed her survival, as compared to the person she shared her room with, to the "valium support system" available to her: "Somehow she [roommate] didn't receive as much loving. Though she appeared more robust than I, she faded away and died. Nurses are more or less valium figures. Roommate was fed, washed and groomed as often as I, but when she was touched, she screamed and cursed; nurses were antagonized."[47] Roommate yearned for McGill's friends. What is crucial, to return to Sloterdijk's use of the citation from Jean Paul, is that McGill undertook the work of writing under the sign of love and friendship to underwrite loving friendship: letters as "telecommunication in the medium of print to underwrite friendship." To underwrite is a pledge, a guarantee, in the case of loss. Who was underwriting whose loss? McGill's letters were a demand for a guarantee, whose etymological root (French: *guarir*) means to protect or defend, a request for protection, as well as its own proof, expressed through her own account of the warrant, the justification for such protection, her writing hence also underwriting itself, in addition to being a call to another. Hence her insistence on, her worry about, the reasonableness of her demands and her concern with being unreasonable.

Repeatedly it returned as a preoccupation, which we saw already with Dr. Reider: Were her demands reasonable? What could she expect in terms of valium? One of the nurses, Mitchell, who appeared to have attended carefully to McGill, often said that McGill is "spoiled rotten," saying it as she brushes her hair softly or feeds her ice cream: "I am not sure just how to respond. Although she [Mitchell] shows me great attention whenever her time and energy permit and is largely responsible for my present good health, 'spoiled rotten' has unpleasant connotations for me. It connotes unreasonable demands, temper tantrums, perpetual crying, etc. I don't think that is an accurate description of my behavior, though some of my efforts to communicate might be interpreted that way by those who don't know me well."[48] McGill wrote that for her, "spoiled" means "the person who clings and screams in terror"; to be spoiled, in her terms, is less about the action received, the caress, than the excessive demand found in the "behavior of an anxiety-ridden and frightened person."[49] She did not pursue the point, which necessarily links the two sides, that of the call and the action in return.

Suffice it to recall the following, something that she wrote in the early months of her hospitalization: "When one's identity is diminished to near zero, and one's energy is near minus and one is confined to a bed in the same room day after day, one's perspective changes, and everything seems to revolve around one's pain and anxiety and lost hopes. So it was that I could believe that all overheard conversations were about me, and all countenances expressed feelings emanating from attitudes toward me. So the whole world revolves around me. I was almost as innocent as a new born baby in this respect."[50] Almost. Babies cannot be innocent to the extent that we cannot attribute guilt to them: they make their needs known, received as demands, and under normal circumstances, babies do not give up on their call to be attended to. McGill is endeavoring to approach her strained relationship with having to make a sound, in lieu of recognizable speech, to make her demand heard. Hence, she could write regarding the "most valium nurses," of whom, crucially and not incidentally, were both nurses who did not "speak code," one, Nurse Molly Keizer, "though she doesn't understand code, she understands my needs almost always . . . I feel safe, secure and sane in her presence."[51] Writing of the meticulous procedure Nurse Keizer followed for turning her on her side, McGill noted that most nurses first set up pillows, then turned her, then stuffed an extra pillow under her head, asking is she is comfortable, by which point, after having been turned and jostled, her head and feet had been moved out of place, leaving her in discomfort for several hours: "Unless I fuss, they aren't inclined to note. If I fuss, I reinforce my spoiled brat image. While they fume in exasperation, I fuss because that is my only way of saying that things aren't right. If I don't call their attention to my discomfort, I may be miserable for the next four or five hours."[52] Valium was her name for being able to avoid being spoiled, which is to say, to avoid having to put into a call her demand to respond to her discomfort. Valium as pleasure.

There is then a second aspect to her "valium support," or rather an aspect of such support as pleasure that points beyond the pleasure of not having to say or do anything in order to be comfortable, to be maintained qua physical body. There is an "enjoyment" that McGill encounters, which like valium goes around or obviates speech, but like the problematic demand is experienced as "excess," the enjoyment of her labile affect caused by ALS, pseudobulbar affect. Lieberman and Benson's paper, published off the back of what I have supposed were Lieberman's meetings with McGill, published under the title "Control of Emotional Expression in Pseudobulbar Palsy," quotes from McGill's writings, without naming her directly. They cite her, as in her letters, writing of the "valium" of the first sight of her son when he comes to visit her: "I often begin laughing at the sight of him . . . first that disturbed me as being altogether crazy, but now I understand it better. The sight of him pleasures me. It gives me joy. I am laughing for joy. And although I would wish I had more sensible and controlled reaction, since I can't seem to help it, I might as well enjoy it."[53] Gazing on her son within her voicelessness.

She wrote to her Dear People that without their vast valium support, she too would have been diminishing: "In fact, I am nothing without all of you." If valium points to the pleasure of not having to cry out and the excess of pleasure as a kind of enjoyment, there is, then, a last aspect to account for, namely, her drive to put this experience into words.

The Body of the Text, the Text of Her Body

Writing was the medium of her demand and the mark of her continuing to exist, the proof of that existence and of that demand, to the extent that writing is an *act*, in the strong sense of requiring "reading" and "interpretation" and even "interpreters," the valium-medium through which she could avoid the creature's call, so as to be able to put demand into a voice, even if it is not, especially because it is not, her own. Writing allowed her to enjoy an act that knots together the physical reality of her body, its capacities, the work she conducted on her loss in the register of her image, and the symbolic work in terms of valium and flaking, the separation of her self and the experience to which she is subject. She appears to have enjoyed the work, however, aside from, sometimes in spite of, the interpretive requirement. Pride: A shadow, or a reflection, of her loss? "I take great pride in these Dear People letters, even though I admit that they are not literary masterpieces and not great entertainment either, nor do they contain much wisdom; but they're my own creations, and each letter, each word, each thought is painstakingly either dictated or written by my eyes and head."[54] With pride comes a fall. A key valium figure, aside from nurses ("more or less" valium), is a rabbi whom she first met when he came into her room at Rosh Hashana and blew the shofar;[55] she was delighted. He often came to see McGill after that, to read to her and to talk to her. By the time of her encounter with the rabbi, McGill was writing in two ways: the first way was through the use of Morse code and the patient assistance and labor of her friend Mary Mae, her son Paul, and her paid "interpreter"; the second way was using the "Tufts Interactive Communicator" (TIC) machine, which had arrived, finally, in April 1977.

McGill sent a letter to the rabbi, as "thanks for valium," and to respond to some of the topics and themes about which he had spoken to her, written using code and her scribes. The next time he saw her, he praised the "interpretations of Mary Mae and Thomascine," which bruised her pride (it "hurt"). She clarified her practice:

> My interpreters, like good secretaries, take dictation in Morse Code. They are remarkable for their patience and devotion. These letters are not written by telepathy or intuition; they take hours of hard work. The Morse Code can be found in most dictionaries. The letter "A" is ".-" or, in my case, "door/window," or "right/left." The word "can" is "-.-./.-/-." The interpreters have to watch my head and eye movements as I spell, and spell out each word—a long tedious process difficult to describe fully. But the advent of the TIC machine seemed to present a means of demonstrating the procedure.[56]

The TIC would be her chance to show the rabbi that the words are her own: "Alas, the TIC takes even longer for to write with than the code. Although it does give an instant transcription in familiar letters, figures and symbols like a typewriter, a scanlight has to search 56 squares, first vertically and then horizontally, and I have to tap the headswitch twice during the double scan to identify the letter or symbol, and unfortunately I am not dexterous nor agile with my head."[57] She wanted to show the rabbi how she could write, that her "interpreters" were actually transcribers, not translators. She wrote him a note, responding to a couple of topics from his visits, and she included a note at the end to explain the machine and technique she was using to write to him. She added a line to the note to explain what he should do if he should catch her in the process of writing: "I asked him to enter and stand beside me, facing the TIC screen, and to wait until this sign, '-/-' appeared on the screen to indicate I was ready for conversation."[58] McGill narrates the story of the first encounter after he received this note and these instructions, a slapstick fall. The rabbi entered her room and saw her in the process of writing on the TIC. He waited as instructed for her to be ready, at which point she gave the sign.

"Well, I guess you expect to answer me back now, don't you?"

"Yes," typed McGill.

The rabbi then "leaned compassionately against the bed rail to watch the screen for more. This act caused the head-switch to jam against my head and wedged me into an immovable condition."[59] She could not move enough to tap, and after several minutes of waiting, looking at the screen, he stood up straight and went to look at the text on the tape coming out of the back of the TIC machine.

"Remarkable! How do you do it Frances?"

She joyously tapped, "hard concentra." Seeing her at work tapping, he came around to her side and began leaning on the bed rail again, bringing her movements and her words to a halt. Her bodily enjoyment and enjoyment of speech were, here with the TIC machine as with the use of Morse code by way of her eyes, literally linked. The difference being that the TIC machine is a self-sufficient medium for the production of letters, not requiring the observation of another human being. It is precisely this self-sufficient medium of speech subsequently received by an other that produced the possibility of misunderstanding: not understanding why she had stopped writing, the rabbi tried to create a sense for what he saw on the screen, which became not an answer to his question about how she is able to "do it," instead reading "hard contentra" as a statement, a demand, reading that she was saying "that it is hard for her to concentrate," to which he then responded to his own reading of what he imputed to her: "All right, Frances, I will leave you to concentrate!"

She wrote, later in a letter, that she was "crestfallen." "Torn between tears of mortification and helpless giggles, I decided that it served me right for wanting to show off."[60] Mortification and helpless giggles: a precipitate of experience in words. Indeed, McGill made the link between bodily enjoyment and writing explicit, by way of an association with what she observed around her, the normative injunctions that she drew out of the interactions between patients who have come to spend their last days and months, and sometimes, as with McGill, years, at the hospital, and the staff, particularly around the dying body and the use of pleasure: "Dying old ladies should say their prayers, not swear. Grown men don't whimper. Old men have no right to masturbate and dream. If an old woman dares to emulate him and do a bit of dreamy masturbation, too, she becomes the object of scorn and ridicule."[61] McGill's case in point is Annie, aged ninety, who had suffered a series of strokes and whose only family were several nieces who sometimes visited her. Annie enjoyed two things: eating and masturbating, the latter for which she was constantly interrogated and even restrained, wrists tied to the bed. Turning her gaze on her self, McGill writes, "Dying is hard, ugly and debasing. I try to celebrate each passing moment of life as best I can. Like a mad musician, I assemble a host of words and phrases and build them into grand symphonic masterpieces; or that is how I fantasize as I tap away at my TIC machine. I affirm life. So, too, did Annie—in her own way."[62] This affirmation occurs through the work of "trying to keep the most live and precious parts of me together, intact: memory, imagination, senses, what wits I have, love or the ability to relate to others."[63] The trope that emerges is one of hope, a hope, though, for "escape," for death, a hope that will, necessarily, be fulfilled: "People who must mark time in a hospital until life's end have a great need for hope of escape from the pain and despair, the terror and tedium, and the outrage to ego and personhood that are part of the prolonged terminal experience."[64] Her deliverance can be located in the contrast between marking time and the time of the letter. She was often frustrated in her daily writing with technical problems, interferences, a bad day for the interpreter, and so on. Sometimes, though, "I feel a surge of joyous excitement and begin to soar as I hope that I have been able to express my thoughts well enough to catch fire in another's mind and heart. When sharing like that happens, I have a feeling of near perfection despite all my limitations. Even while my body is slowly dying, I soar in aliveness as I write. 'O, Didn't My Lord Deliver Daniel?!' I have been delivered, certainly, over and over again."[65] While her body was dying, she soared in aliveness. Sometimes. Experientially, here, dying indexes "that I can no longer move my arms or legs nor roll or twist my body in any way. Save for my head, my body is an inert mass that digests, excretes, breathes, sweats, and experiences sensations of discomfort and pain etc."[66] She had little to no control over her mouth and tongue. She could not inhale, exhale, cough, or blow at will. Her gag reflex was gone. Air went in with food, and she relied on the cough reflex not to choke. And she could tell us this, by writing; soaring in aliveness as she writes against the dying of the light.

PLEA FOR A BLESSING

January 2020. After six months in ALS and palliative care clinics, I wanted, for the time that remained for fieldwork, which I had thought would be until June, to meet and talk with people diagnosed with ALS, outside of clinic, ideally at home. I had left information leaflets with the people I met in the clinic, asking them to contact me if they were open to the idea of me visiting them at home. No one got in touch. After several weeks, at the beginning of February, I asked in both clinics whether they had anyone specific in mind who they thought might be open to talking to me: I compiled a list of about six names, and one name came up immediately in both clinics: Emma. Pia was the first to mention her: a character, charming, one of a kind, direct, a county sheriff, and she liked to talk; Pia thought she would say yes. So did Sylvie, at palliative care. I was sitting in the palliative care office, and I remarked that Pia had given me the same name. A few weeks previously, Emma had requested medical aid in dying, Sylvie explained. Her request had been accepted. Ever ready to act, Sylvie went straight to the phone and called Emma. "She lives in Petaluma, chicken country," she said, as she waited for Emma to pick up. Sylvie chatted a little, checking in to see how Emma was doing, and explained that there was a British anthropologist who was interested in talking to her. Sylvie passed me the phone. Immediately I realized that it would be easier to discern the words Emma was saying if I could see her face. I explained that I wanted to talk with people diagnosed with ALS, and we agreed on a day and time. Sylvie apologized once I had hung up, saying she should have warned me it would be hard to understand her.

Through the dryness of San Rafael and onward through Marin, then Sonoma, to the city of Petaluma. Emma had retired there from San Francisco, where she had worked as a San Francisco County sheriff deputy for twenty-four years, finishing her service in 2018. Emma lived in a prefabricated housing complex of one-story homes, tidy greens, and smooth roads, just across the way from her friend and former boss Shaleen. Her home was fitted with a mechanical lift to get up to the entrance. Dogs barked as I rang the bell in the heat of midday. The doormat stated "Come as you are." The person who opened the door surprised me, her movements perfectly slow: Emma was large, a physically soft face and a gaze that did not hold back, and as we shook hands, I felt scrutinized. She was wearing a cap that said NRA on it, which I supposed meant National Rifle Association. I decided it was not ironic, although I have my doubts.

Less than a year after retiring and moving, Emma broke her arm while changing a lightbulb. She fell off the ladder. She went into the hospital with a broken arm. She came out of the hospital ten weeks later with a diagnosis of ALS. She told me that when she went in, she was supposed to have surgery on her arm, but the anesthesiologist said that if he put her under general anesthetic, he would not be able to extubate her: "I don't know why. I didn't ask the right questions at the time." She was diagnosed with asthma and chronic obstructive pulmonary disease (COPD) as well. This was in May 2019. By the time of our meeting, nine months later, the family and friends that had initially been present and who had been more than willing to help were "burned out." She told me she was afraid. Sitting perpendicular to her, intensely watching her face to make sure I could catch the sounds and then the words she was saying, I did not ask of what. She then asked me if I believe in God. I said something about having been baptized as a child. She shot back that I had not answered her question. "It's a blessing," she then said, returning to her illness, "I'm supposed to learn something from it."

There were things that she already knew: she would not accept invasive ventilation or the feeding tube, just as her brother had not wanted to accept such tools for the prolongation of a bodily existence. Their father and grandfather both had had tracheotomies. She had had to intervene for her brother, a long time ago, when he died with AIDS. He had made his wishes clear: "no extraordinary measures." The hospital team had given him a "full code" once his body began to fail, despite his prior plea. A tracheotomy was done and he was put on ventilation. She would do everything she could to make it right. As Emma told me this, she ran her finger along the table in front of her: "I was on a line, this side I was losing my mind, this side, I didn't want my brother to die." In the hospital room, she was about to leave to go outside to smoke a cigarette. As she reached the door, she saw two angels land on each of her brother's shoulders: "this is the time, this is the time," she told the team, and she was the one to switch off the machine that was keeping his body alive: "I saw a light with *sparkledust*, his soul leaving his body." She was very close to her brother. There were other siblings, but he was the one she was close to. They were wards of the state, growing up in "LA-laland." They had been taken away from their parents. It was too soon to know why.

I asked Emma about how she takes care of herself and who is able to help out: a nurse comes twice a week; she also has social worker who visits as well as physical therapy once a week. She told me that she made a request for aid in dying. She had heard about it and looked it up. There was no hope in clinical trials: too old, or else the illness was too advanced already. "I pray that God will help me to know when is the right time." She said that she still had things to sort out and to work through. "If you don't understand me, say something, don't just nod," she said, with a serious look. I was on the spot, of course, it was a test, and so I said back to her the words I had just heard. I thought that with this stern injunction, addressed to me, she was also telling herself not to give up. "The problem is you don't know what is next, what part of the body and how severe it will be." I waited. "You look so sad," she said.

Poor Me Syndrome

The next time I went to see Emma was about two weeks later, in mid-February; I sent her a text message the day prior to our meeting. I was worried, I think, that I would get there, knock on the door, and find that she had died. She didn't reply. She was there, however. Her mood, though, was different. The first time I met her, I had felt a very sudden, strong attachment, a mutuality of feeling, I liked her; I could see she liked the contact with me. I got a big hug before I had left, and she made me promise that I would say hello to Pia from her; she clearly enjoyed the thought that I spent time in clinic with her, Pia, her "favorite person" at clinic. This time, she was clearly very low, very sad, and I think was wary of having to talk to me again.

She asked me what my questions were. I began to say something, and she began to cry. It's getting harder for people to understand her, she said. Her face slowly broke out from a gaze focused toward me into a sobbing wail directed to an elsewhere. I recognized the facial gesture of her tears as the kind of "crumbling" and collapse of which Frances McGill wrote. Emma got up, walked slowly away, and eventually came back. When she sat down again, she smiled at me through the veil of her tears.

What do I want to know? I recapped what we spoke about the last time, and I told her that I wanted to know more about her request for medical aid in dying, given the work I had already done in Switzerland, which I told her a little bit about. I had gone to a California conference on "medical aid in dying," which I had told her about the last time, and she had said that she wanted to know more about how it actually works here in California, and so I told her what I had heard. As I spoke, I noticed a change in affect, from down and forlorn to a sort of neutral attentiveness, something to focus on, an object of attention: I wrote down several points that I thought were important to be aware of, notably, to make sure the hospice nursing team knew about her plans, and if possible for someone to be on hand, to assist the family should something unexpected occur, notably a concern regarding patients who will take longer than four hours to die after ingestion of the medical aid in dying drugs. Emma asked whether she has to be able to swallow the liquid, which I confirmed, or else, to use a device to administer the solution through the rectum, which would likely need to be supervised by a nurse, or health professional, or in the event that she had a feeding tube, it could be administered through that—although it is unlikely any clinic would accept to put in a feeding tube if they knew the main reason for the patient was to use it as a way of ending their life.

One key issue practitioners are concerned about is the occurrence of prolonged time to death, after ingestion (anything over four or five hours). The major cause is paresis of the gut, such that the medication cannot get into the duodenum. To do medical aid in dying, Emma would have to be enrolled in hospice; there should be communication with the prescribing doctor and the palliative care team that has been following her; there is the question of who will be present, who will take responsibility for mixing the medication, and that she should be aware of the possibility, even though remote, that something could go wrong, and hence there should be a plan B in place, which would be palliative sedation until death, organized by the hospice nursing team.

All of this technical discussion was clearly relieving to both of us. I was in a position of knowing something. I was soon to disappoint.

"Why did I get this illness?" she asked.

"Nobody can answer that question, in your case," I replied. A tiny minority of ALS cases are of genetic origin. For everyone else, there is a hole in knowledge.

There is nothing to be done, she told me: she was too old for stem cell trials, she couldn't take medication for emotional lability because it interferes with heart medication she was taking, and she didn't want to talk to palliative care over the phone because she feared no one would understand her. She asked me not to say anything about her to the palliative care team. Her next ALS clinic appointment was at a satellite clinic in Santa Rosa, the county capital twenty miles north; her friend Helen would take her. I told her I would see her there. "Does everyone cry as much as I do?" she asked me. "I have poor me syndrome."

She said that she really hopes Pia will be at clinic. "Tell her that I said you're a meanie for making me cry."

Is This the Time?

The satellite clinic is run out of a university building in a medical facilities strip mall in Santa Rosa. Most of the time, it functions as a pediatric and gynecological cancer clinic. A few colleagues told me that Emma had not confirmed her appointment and that they hoped I was not wasting my time. I had a feeling she would show up. It was March 13, 2020. A pandemic had been announced two days earlier. All nonessential research was supposed to be stopped: I asked for advice from the clinic director, who told me she considered that I was a part of the team, and so I should be fine to continue coming to clinic. The rooms were filled with the scent of squirt after squirt of hydroalcoholic gel.

I knew from the day before that Pia, the speech and language pathologist, was not coming; it would be Angela: given what I'd been told about Angela, whom Pia replaced at the main clinic, I was curious to meet her. I had been told that affectively it was very hard for her to work with patients with ALS, that she got too involved with patients, and that she took her work home with her and didn't set boundaries.

"It's one o'clock," someone said, "it looks like Emma is not coming." I was talking to Moira about Mrs. Liu, asking how she was doing. She told me that she had gone to her house recently, changed the settings on her ventilator, and had spent about an hour with the family. "She's doing great," Moira said.

"Here she is!" A couple of people exclaimed in chorus. Emma had arrived.

I went out to see her, and met Helen, her friend. Helen had worked at the San Francisco General Hospital, the city's public hospital, for thirty years: she had volunteered to work on the AIDS ward, during the early 1980s, at a time when it still wasn't known how it was transmitted.

Georgina took Emma's vitals, and we walked through into the little exam room. The respiratory specialists came in, Moira and Colette.

"How are you doing?" Colette asked.

"Good days and bad days." Colette didn't say anything and Emma followed up, "Did you understand me?"

"Yeah, I can understand you," Colette replied stiffly. "O2 sat of 88 is kind of her baseline," Colette says to Moira, *beep beep*, "good it went up, 90. Short of breath?"

"Yeah, I'd say so."

"On a scale of one to ten?"

"Three."

"On exertion?"

"Maybe a five."

"Did you bring your mask?"

"No," Emma then made a face at me, mocking them.

"Remember this one? Three breaths: in out in out in; then pause; then blow it out."

As usual, I could not bear to look: it is hard enough to do this, without everyone looking at you. Emma did it.

"What is it?"

"Twenty-eight."

"What should it be?"

"Sixty. So your numbers are a little on the lower side. Test two is the one where you suck in. Twenty percent exactly like last time."

"Can you make a seal with your lips?"

"Yeah."

"Oh, that looks pretty good. Now we're going to put a clip on your nose, you'll exhale, inhale, then blow out. Twenty-nine percent, one more time. Eleven percent. Did you feel like your throat tightened up? That one won't count. You have to blow fast enough for the machine to record."

"Well that is why I'm here. I tried my best."

"Let's see if we get anything. . . . Twenty-one percent."

"Let's do one more, that you blow hard. Are you tired?"

"I'm tired of this!" Emma gave a look halfway between a scowl and grin. "It closes off," she said, referring to her throat.

"That's laryngospasm. Best peak flow 97 liters per minute. Twenty-seven percent FVC. Are you able to cough?" Emma coughed. "So that's a no. Do you have a cough assist?"

"I used it yesterday."

"How many times a day do you use it?"

"Three."

"How many breaths do you do?"

"Five cycles three times a day."

"You have phlegm? What color is it?"

"Lately it's been clear."

"Swallowing?"

"I want to say no, but I choke a little, on watermelon."

"Have you lost weight?"

"164 today," Emma said not answering the question.

"Sleep?"

"I wake up in the middle of the night."

"Are you okay? Your lips turned purple. You weren't breathing."

"I wasn't doing it on purpose."

There was panic in the room and Moira quickly went to get some oxygen. Eventually Moira got a mask onto Emma's face, and she started to look a little better. Moira asked how she is feeling. Typically, oxygen therapy alone is not provided for patients with ALS except as part of so-called comfort care, because delivery of oxygen alone can suppress respiratory drive and lead to worsening hypercapnia. In Emma's case, it was indicated because of her comorbidities.

"Has it been any better since you started with the oxygen therapy?"

"I didn't like it at first, but then we became friends."

The respiratory therapists asked questions about her service provider for her machines, whether there was anything she'd like to change in terms of settings, and then said goodbye to Emma, leaving Helen, Emma, and me in the room.

James the dietician entered the room.

"You're losing weight, 164 and some change."

"Sometimes I'm just not hungry. Tired of chewing and chewing. So I just stop."

"Are we talking about hamburgers?"

"Oh no, hamburgers go down just fine."

Helen intervened to say that Emma gets food delivered.

"Whole Foods. Four entrees, once a week."

"How many meals a day is that?"

"Between none and three."

"You're still snacking in the middle of the night? I remember you don't sleep well."

"Blueberries with whipped cream. Fresh fruit."

"If we can, it would be good to get your weight up."

"I want to lose weight."

"Why?"

"I want to be able to tie my shoes. I want to get down to 140. Why don't you want me to lose weight? It's ironic the two skinniest people in the room are telling me to put on weight."

"It will affect your breathing. If you lose weight, you'll go quicker."

While James was looking down at his notepad writing, Emma looked over at me and stuck two fingers in her mouth to make a vomiting gesture. She found her joke hilarious. James caught a glimpse of the gesture and decided to wrap the session up.

"Look, I just want to encourage you to eat, for it to be pleasurable, I see you with your legs crossed, you can tie your shoes fine. Plus it's going to be harder to tie your shoes at 140 [pounds] than it is now."

"I'm going to eat more salad."

"If you do that, lots of dressings, cut avocado."

"I love avocado. If I wouldn't feed it to my dog, I won't eat it."

"Does your dog eat avocado? And tomorrow is pie day, you *have to* have a pie on pie day." He left.

Angela the speech pathologist came in and told Emma that they had met before, once, when Emma was in the hospital, just after her diagnosis. She said that "they had a moment."

"I don't remember, I don't want to lie, and add that to the list," Emma said, pointing upward.

Angela showed Emma a little note from Pia. Emma told Angela about how she calls Pia "meanie."

"She's usually the softy. I'm the hard one! Based on Pia's notes, is it true that sometimes you are including other ways of communicating? Using your boogey board?"

"Not using it. I don't want to lie."

Angela somewhat apologetically says she doesn't think she has anything new for Emma. She said she wants to focus on alleviating as much as possible the stress that comes with trying to communicate. Other patients who use multiple modalities often find they have better communication. Usually we understand about 90 percent; then, in order to get one or two words, you can use a support, instead of having to go back to the beginning.

"Any other questions about communications?"

Emma begins to say something, then begins to cry. "I miss being part of it," she said. Once she calmed herself a bit, Emma asked Angela if she was using sign language.

"No, it's just how I talk, using my hands."

Helen clarified that Emma is a proficient speaker of sign language. Angela explained that there are tools like Assistive Express, which would work well with an iPad, and indicated that there may be a state aid program to help with paying for a device. She went out to find out if this is possible.

The occupational therapist Jess was next to see Emma. They discussed her pain, which has increased a lot, and how the home is set up and how she is doing in terms of mobility and feeding herself. Jess asked if Emma would consider a hospital bed. Emma said something, which Jess did not understand. Nor did Helen. Emma considered repeating herself and then waved her hand as though to say "forget about it." I thought I had understood, so reluctantly I intervened:

"Is this the time?" I said.

Emma smiled. I added an interpretation of the statement, that I had understood that it meant, if she wants the hospital bed, does she have to say so right now. Jess clarified that she can put in the request now, which is valid for three months, and all that would then be needed is for a doctor to put in the order.

It was significant to me that I had heard her question, "Is this the time?"

Dr. Ackerman was the last person to see Emma. Her clinic so far had taken about four hours. Emma and Helen looked pretty drained.

"I know you had a long day. You followed up with palliative care. What's bothering you?"

"A lot of back pain. Missed a dose of morphine, woke up in a lot of pain."

"MS contin [morphine] as base pain medication, gabapentin for neuropathic pain, and opioids for breakthrough pain?"

Helen added that Emma had oxycodone, an opioid, but she kept falling. She has not taken it since December.

"Might be a good idea?"

"I won't take it again."

Dr. Ackerman and Emma had a discussion with respect to Emma's concern about which team is in charge, ALS or palliative care, and who is making the decisions. Emma asked what is the role of each doctor; she said that from her point of view, they are just kicking the ball to one another. How to manage her pain? How to be able to speak better? Is the pain from ALS or something else?

"When I first got diagnosed, they said a year and half, well I'm still here."

Her physical examination showed that strength in her legs hadn't changed. Her speech problems are connected to her weight loss. She tells the doctor she has loss of appetite.

"Not like the food they used to have in the Castro, eh!" Dr. Ackerman said, referring to the neighborhood in San Francisco where Emma used to live as a young sheriff.

"It's not fun being told what to eat."

"How is your mood?"

"I hate the evil sisters."

Dr. Ackerman diplomatically stated that respiratory therapy is not always comfortable and that she is sure the therapists are doing their upmost to make Emma feel comfortable, and if there are any specific concerns that Emma has, she'll pass on any constructive criticism.

"I can't stop crying."

"Yes, there is definitely PBA [pseudobulbar affect], but it's mainly depression. Could we switch your antidepressant? For example, Remeron; it's also an appetite stimulant. Have you ever been overweight?"

"I've weighed more than I weigh now. I feel comfortable, less pain."

"I hear that, but the weight loss is accelerating the disease."

Dr. Ackerman took the occasion mentioning that Emma's illness is accelerating to say that she wanted to talk to Emma about end-of-life options: "Have you talked to palliative care about other ways of dying? Some people have milestones or redlines; for others, it's more of a gray zone; even before EOLOA [End of Life Option Act], there were lots of ways to help people die peacefully."

Helen clarified that once Emma goes on hospice, no one else will come to the house.

"That is true but hospice sends a nurse, overseen by a physician, and they do intensive symptom management. It gets to a point where we ask what are your primary goals? My goals for you: better mood; more quality awake time; enjoying your friends and family. I think maybe hospice could give you more benefit than physical therapy and occupational therapy."

Emma agreed to look into hospice.

"It looks to me that it is mainly pain and existential suffering. I see someone who is suffering more than they need to be."

"When can I see you again?"

"In a month in a televisit."

"If I'm on hospice, will you still take care of me?"

"Yes."

The Time Was Coming

Emma died two months later in May. I spoke to her briefly once on the phone, after seeing her at the clinic, through FaceTime, and she sent me Easter wishes in April. The disruption of the pandemic was only partly the reason I did not go to see her again. After the last clinic visit, the talk of hospice, it was clear she knew the time was coming and that she had work to do, spiritual and theological work, not anthropological work, so to speak. I came to hear about Emma's last two months from the palliative care chaplain, Dr. Lange, who had recently joined the clinic. Dr. Lange had gotten to know Emma in the last six weeks of her life, at first during a palliative care telehealth visit, which was heavily focused on managing her symptoms, and then Dr. Lange had started speaking with her weekly after that, "following a moment of huge spiritual distress that just bubbled up through her being," the chaplain said.

Dr. Lange narrated to me what she understood about the things Emma was going through, what she was trying to work through, in that period following her last clinic visit: when they began to talk regularly, she had just gone through a period of deep depression, which corresponded to a period directly following her last clinic visit. Dr. Lange linked the period of depression and Emma's thoughts about her illness to experiences that she had had as a child, growing up as a ward of the state of California. She had been taken from her parents as a child because her parents were deaf. She went to live with her aunt, which was when she began to attend an evangelical church. The aunt with whom she went to live, from the time that Emma was a child, had apparently made statements to Emma that there was something sinful about her, connected to questions of sexuality. The chaplain described what she took to be "a lot of transference and countertransference" in the encounter between herself and Emma, turning on the fact that they are both lesbian women, and she drew on that to try and unpack how perceptions of her homosexuality as a child, by her caregivers, in relation to this spiritual community that her aunt introduced her to, was knotted to language around "innate sinfulness." Emma described "hearing stories of Jesus at that time, and as having a deep feeling that there was this kind man who loved children and that he loved her, and she knew that somehow in her body, and at the same time what was being said in a way that wasn't being located in anything specific, that there was something deep inside that was bad. And that was connected to faith and to Jesus."

Emma, I was told, had become very stuck and worried in her discussions with the chaplain about purgatory. "When we first met, one of the things she was fearful about was going to hell, she wanted to know if hell existed, what could send you there. Interestingly, I thought at first I was trying to assess whether it was related to the medical aid in dying choice she was making, because many people have that question. And that did not seem to be the case with her, it was something else." Emma had frequently repeated to me, likewise, that she did not consider her decision to request medical aid in dying a sin, saying, "He would understand."

The core concerns, in the chaplain's view, were of self-worth and belonging, sinfulness and this specific worry about purgatory. "So Emma was very worried about where she was going to go when she died and she was worried about who would be there and who would not be there. Her theology very clearly included a heaven and a hell and her feeling was that when you got at least to heaven, you would see people you loved who were there, and she wanted to know, which I found so sweet, and telling, she's so relational, she wanted to know, at least if she went to purgatory, would the people that she knew and loved and didn't make the cut for heaven, whether they'd be there."

The chaplain had wondered whether Emma's concerns about belonging and this deep feeling of innate sinfulness, and the worry about where she would "go," were tied to a history of a person who "never came out" about their sexuality. Dr. Lange was thus surprised to learn from Emma that she was very much off the mark: Emma had very much been part of a lesbian community in San Francisco in the 1970s and 1980s and after. I had wondered whether Emma's brother was gay, given that they had a particularly close relationship, and from the chronology, I had assumed he had died in the early 1980s. Dr. Lange's narrative about her work with Emma was assisting me certainly not in "understanding" Emma but at least to specify elements that could give some orientation, some coordinates, for aspects of the way she talked about her symptoms: the fact that she was taken away from her parents because they were deaf: I can only speculate that the signification of having lost the capacity to be understand through speech, from ALS, is tied to the separation she underwent from her parents with whom she had a very particular form of communication that did not rely on sound. They could talk without sound, something clearly lacking with the rest of us.

As the chaplain and Emma worked together, Emma would go through cycles; "at times it would be questions of hell and purgatory," and at other times, it would be a spiritual quest to open something up in her relation to God, "and then she had a spiritual experience, a very direct spiritual experience," a few weeks before her death, one of "really feeling she was reconciled to God." It was this experience that ended the period of depression: "It was the first time that I perceived her as not being so fearful of lack of connectedness. And that was the first time she talked to me about her death not as a kind of abrupt moment, and more of a transition, and she had a very different relationship to it after that."

Emma described the event of this reconciliation as coming out of "deep depression but not really depression because it was about important things." She came to the realization that she would not be alone spiritually as she neared and experienced death. Her fear of being outside of grace, a key characteristic of her Christian faith, had subsided, and her concern with going to hell was replaced for Emma by a deep sense of knowing from God that she is loved by Jesus and is not and will never be abandoned by him.

Dr. Lange said that they reflected on the wisdom that Emma had as a little girl when she would attend Sunday school and hear stories about "a nice man who loved everyone." Dr. Lange asked Emma if she ever spoke to that little girl, and she said that she has been "trying to connect to her more and more these days." Dr. Lange told of how she coached Emma in practices through which she could cultivate this loving connection to her younger self and draw on the strength and insight she gleans from it, as well as how Emma reflected on the peace she felt, but emphasized that she would "need her spiritual teachers around her for this part of the journey." Dr. Lange recounted how Emma told her that their work together had "opened a portal for her to get back to God."

Time Is Out of Joint

Emma did not talk to Dr. Lange during this period of theological–spiritual work, roughly from March 23 to May 6, about her choice or the timing of her request for medical aid in dying. It was on a palliative care telehealth visit on May 6 that she shared with the team that she felt that it was time, "the time was coming," and she ordered the medication. "And even at that time I did not understand that she meant to do it so quickly. It was very surprising to me." Dr. Lange asked her what brought her to make the request for the medication, expecting a theological answer, whereas what Emma replied was that felt she was losing her independence. It was becoming very clear to Emma that she would not be able to care for herself for much longer, that it was becoming more difficult to communicate.

Helen had gone to visit her for the weekend with another friend, Doreen; they went on Saturday, May 9. Emma decided on the Saturday that it was going to be in the next few days that she would take the aid in dying medication. First she picked Tuesday, then Wednesday, as the day to take the lethal medication, the day to die.

While discussing which day to choose, Emma realized that she was about to run out of pain medication. So before picking the date, she made sure that the day she picked was on the day when she'd have access to it. The chaplain said to me that she found it hard to understand as a way of thinking about which day to choose to die. She went so far as to say that she even wondered whether cognitively Emma was okay or not: "That was where it was weird to me, like is this person making sense. I could understand wanting to do it because you don't want to go through all day Monday in pain, although I don't think that's a reason to end your life, but that's not my judgment, but why did she want to do it on the day the pain meds were being delivered? I asked her if she was worried they won't be strong enough if she'd need backup pills, and she laughed and said, I'm not telling anyone."

Regardless of Emma's reasoning and of Dr. Lange's confusion, this point was a very literal confirmation of knowledge drawn from work on assisted suicide, which indicates that people don't do assisted suicides in order to avoid pain. It's an action that occurs on another register. In a certain way, Dr. Lange then echoed this thought: "What she kept coming back to in the last weeks was this feeling of freedom, due to this internal work that she did, something happened where she had a direct experience of acceptance and continuity, that transcended death, of a kind of belonging, that to me was new to her, because up until then, she had not wanted anyone to know that she was going to do this, she didn't want her sisters there, and that changed at the end." In the end, Emma died surrounded by both friends and family.

The plan, which had been drawn up on the Saturday, was for Emma to die on Wednesday. Her niece was informed, and they had a visit all together with the chaplain through Zoom. Dr. Lange was concerned about Emma dying with unfinished business and wanted to help Emma die with a sense of "completion." "And she kept saying, I feel free, I feel free, I feel free, and she was experiencing more and more pain, her symptoms were progressing really quickly, it was getting so hard to understand her, she was getting so tired so quickly, she couldn't even really write anymore and it was really interesting to see that she had this profound healing experience, existential healing experience as her body was unravelling at this time." In that meeting, they were able to plan with Emma what she wanted for the end of her life: the music she wanted, the prayer she wanted, who she wanted to be there.

But Emma did not die on Wednesday.

On Sunday night, she fell badly and was taken by Helen, who was with her, to the emergency room. She wound up really decompensating over the next day. Doreen, the friend who had gone to visit Emma, texted Dr. Lange at 18:49 and said, "Emma is passing, do you want to say goodbye?" The hospice nurse had come, earlier that day. The last time she was awake was at 1 P.M., "and then at a certain point her oxygen was down to 50, and so I was then Face Timed in to give Emma a benediction and a commendation." The chaplain was wondering whether she took the medication in secret, but Emma's friends disconfirmed this. She had, though, stopped using BiPAP two weeks previously.

Helen ended up not leaving on Sunday after Emma came home from the hospital, so she was there, Shaleen was there, as well as another friend, and ultimately Emma's sister appeared. Emma had decided on Saturday that she had wanted to tell her siblings. So on Tuesday morning, Dr. Lange received a text message: Emma was going downhill quickly, her body was letting go. The chaplain learned that Emma had decided to tell her niece and sister so that they could come to see her if they wanted to. "It was very dramatic," the chaplain said, narrating what happened as Emma's sister entered the scene: *Emm wake up wake up look at me, you can't die.* There was still more to be said, at least for her. She was out of time.

ADVOCATE

Nathan buzzed me into the apartment, from somewhere downtown, using his phone. He was at the office. It was six weeks before most people, all but essential workers, would stop leaving their homes to go to work, following the unprecedented shelter-in-place order that was to be announced across California.

I had come to talk with Gwen. The research coordinator at the clinic, Georgina, had put us in touch, having described her as "pro research." Gwen graciously accepted my request to talk with her. It had been difficult to find people willing to speak with me about their experience. She called out from inside the apartment, that I should let myself in. Standing at the far end of their open-plan home, holding a walker, a kind gaze met me as I approached her to introduce myself. We sat at the table. I had my back to a flight of stairs that led to a mezzanine bedroom.

Gwen was diagnosed by Dr. Blumen at age thirty-two, two years previously. Roughly 10 percent of people with ALS are aged under forty-five, often called "young-onset" patients. Gwen spoke first of the phase III trial she was enrolled in, the trial that Mrs. Liu had wanted to be in, named by way of a single word, used throughout the patient and medical community: "BrainStorm."

BrainStorm Cell Therapeutics is the name of a company founded in 2004, whose business plan was based on technology developed at the Michael J. Fox Foundation for Parkinson's Research at Tel Aviv University. In December 2011, BrainStorm conducted a phase I/II trial of the injection of autologous cultured mesenchymal bone marrow stromal cells (MSCs) as a possible treatment for patients with ALS, at both early and progressive stages. This first trial was conducted at Hadassah Hebrew University Medical Center, Jerusalem, in Israel. The results led the company to make an application to the FDA for a new investigational drug status, in 2013, for the autologous MSCs they were seeking to produce under the name "NurOwn" and whose therapeutic benefit was hypothesized to come from the neurotrophic factors (NTFs) these cultured autologous cells were modified to produce. In the NurOwn protocol, patients' own MSCs are harvested through an invasive procedure, via lumbar puncture, and "differentiated to secrete high levels of NTFs using a proprietary technology," in the words of the company's promotional materials. The differentiated MSCs, which Brain-Storm have called "MSC-NTF cells," are then gathered and injected (injected back in, so to speak) into the patient. What the mechanism of repair actually consists of is unknown, but they "may activate neuroprotective and immuno-modulatory pathways," according to BrainStorm.

At the time of the first meeting with Gwen in January 2020, she told me that she had been diagnosed at "a pivotal time," a time that was a pivot in her own life, necessarily a turning point, and, it is hoped, a pivotal moment in the search for better treatments. BrainStorm was, at this time, very much one of the visible strings that patients endeavored to hold on to, a knot to which and in which those who had some hope for a change in prognosis in their lifetime tied themselves.

Shortly after diagnosis, Gwen gathered contact information for the trial, which had an enrollment site at an ALS clinic in the city in which she lived: "It's a phase III double-blind placebo-controlled trial," Gwen specified.

What she didn't yet specify, but that I would come to appreciate little by little, as she talked to me over time, was how there is a tension, a tension that has a particular range of affects tied into it, a tension between a supposed requirement of scientific best practice, namely randomization to placebo, and the ethical and political question of whether there might be other, faster, more generative, more compassionate ways of testing therapeutics, better ways of including people with ALS in trials, when the outcome is certain death.

The phase III trial was eleven and a half months long. Of course, she did not know what she received, whether it was the drug or the placebo: "The data will hopefully be released in the autumn [2020]," she told me. At the time of writing, in October 2021, the data had yet to be unblinded.

During this same period, while enrolled in the BrainStorm trial, during the year up until our first meeting, Gwen had been engaged with a nonprofit organization, I AM ALS. The group was founded at the end of 2018 and has been in the process of developing areas of work, of expertise, and of intervention. Gwen had been working on committees concerned with legislation, community, and "pharma" principally preoccupied with assisting people to have more access to trials. "I have been lucky," she said, "that the disease progression has not been rapid."

I asked Gwen, before finding out more about how she is living with ALS, and more about her political work on ALS, to begin with whether she could tell me about her diagnosis: "The diagnosis itself, it's very overwhelming; getting there was hard work too. Starting in October 2016, my left foot began to drop, which led to falls. I went to a private practice and was diagnosed with low blood pressure and anxiety." Despite Frances McGill's use of the comorbidity as a joke (cf. chapter 6), in Gwen's case, low blood pressure sowed confusion. "I rode that diagnosis for a while." I asked whether she was satisfied with it: "I was not satisfied with that diagnosis; I thought, if only my body could speak. My brain was not connecting with my limbs quickly enough. My extremities were heavily impacted. Walking to work, climbing hills, feeling like I was going to fall. It's tough to describe imbalance . . . the feeling of struggling to cross major intersections because I am not quick enough to make the light. My body is just not responding how it used to. When describing these things, there is no formal test; of course I did MRIs of the brain and spinal cord, but nothing turns up on imaging. I understand in a sense what led to the anxiety diagnosis, but when a patient returns with increasing falls, not getting better, there should be a real call to action." It is only in hindsight that I can underscore that from the beginning of our discussions, Gwen spoke of a call, a call to action, and of speech, speech on behalf of the body. To speak for an other is to act as an advocate: *vŏcāre*, to call; to call upon, summon, invoke; to call together, convoke, and *ad*, the crucial prefix "toward," toward a call, to call together toward something: an orientation to a future.

"Historically I have not had anxiety. I have had previous bouts of depression. I was sent to therapists, my mental health was explored. I was prescribed a very low dose of anxiety medication. Side effects include dizziness; I don't think that it exacerbated the falls, but it didn't help." Had she done any research during this time? "I Google searched, which was scary. Two to three months before diagnosis at clinic in May 2018, my symptoms were strikingly similar to descriptions of ALS. Really bad clonus [involuntary and rhythmic muscle contractions], shaking and twitching. Although my speech wasn't slow at that point, it was becoming harder to get words out. Cognitively I knew I was fine, just my movement was not on par with cognition."

Against the Shrug

Gwen underscored different aspects of the clinic that she found helpful, including the fact that data suggest that going to an ALS clinic improves quality and duration of life, a fact that is frequently mentioned in public presentations of the benefits of multidisciplinary care clinics (cf. part 2). She reminded me, moreover, that the clinic is partly financed through the ALS Association (ALSA), the longest standing ALS association in the United States, founded in 1985, and specifically the hours billed by the social workers for the clinic are paid for by ALSA. At the same time, Gwen indicated that there is criticism from within the community (of patients with ALS) that ALSA's orientation to the stakes of their work and their ultimate commitment is to "make us comfortable until we die." There is a dissatisfaction. There is a demand for more: more action, more urgency, more funding, more trials, more effort, more experimentation, which implies more open trial criteria.

Gwen highlighted how invaluable it is to have information about resources, about trials that are open or will open, available observational studies, and participation in biomarker research. As she put it, "We have identified some genes, some targets, there is still so much to learn about." The issue is a dual-sided one for those diagnosed: first, gaining awareness of what is available as a possible avenue for experimental therapy, including where it is based, and second, the issue of urgency, because most trial criteria include the requirement of being signed up within eighteen months of symptom onset. Delaying diagnosis and false diagnoses, while to a degree understandable since this is a clinical diagnosis made through exclusion (except for the rare cases of genetic variants), nevertheless come with something akin to an opportunity cost, an opportunity loss.

How quickly a patient is diagnosed and how quickly the patient can be hooked into a trial that they consider worth venturing into, with the physical, emotional, and other stakes associated, matters significantly to how the person can be oriented toward the illness.

Such urgency and striving, which Gwen incarnates, is the antithesis of what she called "The Shrug," a term that she indicated was used through the community of people with ALS. It is principally used as a metaphor; doctors and clinicians don't often, I suppose, literally shrug. The Shrug as metaphor stems from the image of a gesture that acknowledges an impotence on the side of the medical corps. I never saw a clinician shrug, yet hearing Gwen talk about The Shrug, I began to ask myself whether I too hadn't succumbed to a figuration of ALS as that kind thing over which no one has any power, a figuration that may or may not be true and that, if true, should not come for free, gratuitously, before having striven to undo it.

In my effort to understand available knowledge of ALS, as a historical process, with its senses of certitude and its indeterminations (part 1 of this book) and the clinical apparatuses for managing the illness (part 2), I postulated, as a condition of countenancing ALS as an object of reflection, the current impossibility of cure, an observation stemming from the variegated responses to the question of what to do when faced with the limits of what medical science can know and do. The Shrug is rooted in this impossibility.

The Shrug, however, does not then mean indifference, or lack of action, but it does mean that at present, for those clinicians who have dedicated their professional lives to diagnosing and supporting those with this illness, despite the desire that subtends the continued search for therapies, there is the bedrock of the real that they touch on a daily basis; that so far, they have been shown to be ultimately powerless to control the degenerative process, a specific, and only one specific, kind of powerlessness.

This powerlessness, as a variant on The Shrug, was expressed poignantly when Nathan and Gwen, many months later, returned to the story of Gwen's diagnosis. Recalling that this was for a second opinion, after an initial diagnosis of orthostatic hypotension and anxiety, made by a private practice neurologist, "Dr. Blumen came into the room two seconds after the residents had left, asks me to say 'It's a sunny day in San Francisco,' and then she looks at me like *this*." The facial expression that Gwen made, if put on the Ekman Facial Action Coding System, would be something like "fearful sadness," accompanied by raised shoulders and upturned palms.

The metaphor of The Shrug and the facial expression of fearful sadness are linked to the degree that the gesture of shrugging and the facial expression of fear are antitheses of aggressiveness (in the case of the gesture of the shrug) and anger (in the case of the emotion of fear). The link, I would argue, between the metaphor Gwen indicated and the facial gesture she saw on being diagnosed is the mark of impotence, a counterconduct to aggressiveness or anger, a facing up to a reality of the incurable, the impossibility of cure. This does not mean, however, the lack of possible action. To the contrary, the question is how the individual conceives action, given a confrontation with the contingency of this impossibility.

Not If but When

The nonprofit organization I AM ALS is a case in point of an effort to transform the very terms through which the illness is discussed: "the question is not if we will find cures for ALS but when" is an enunciation that representatives of the organization repeat. The pointed difference between if and when is dampened depending on who the certitude can be for: in this life or not? The hole in knowledge that anchors The Shrug is bracketed in favor of the not-yet-possible, not yet, but one day.

An answer to the question, in this life or not, is critical. What is also critical is that lacking an answer to this question of the timing of certitude in a cure, there is a corresponding increase in the demand for action: I AM ALS, in just two years of work, developed tools to help better orient people diagnosed with ALS to trials, to participate in discussions of clinical trial standards, to argue in Congress for expanded access, and to financially support biological research.

In April 2019, the cofounder Brian Wallach testified in front of the House Appropriations Subcommittee on Labor, Health and Human Services, Education, and Related Agencies regarding the need for increased funding for ALS research. His first congressional testimony is worth citing at length because it underscores several things: first, that it is a political discourse coming from someone who had worked in the Obama administration, a discourse diagnosing political blockages to adequately funding research, and second, that it is a discourse about science to the degree that his discourse draws on tropes of expectation, which indicate the notion that if it weren't for political impediments, and if conditions can be organized so that research can be well funded, a cure, or at the least proper treatment, will necessarily follow.

> Chairwoman DeLauro, Ranking Member Cole, Members of the Committee, thank you for the opportunity to testify before you today. My name is Brian Wallach . . . today an ALS diagnosis means I will not see my daughters grow up. ALS is currently a death sentence. Not because it cannot be cured. But because we have underfunded the fight against ALS year after year after year. I am here today to ask you to rewrite the ALS story. I am here as a co-founder of I AM ALS, a patient-led, patient-centric movement to defeat ALS. I am here on behalf of my family and the incredible ALS community. To ask you to see us, hear us, and to fully fund our fight so we can finally defeat ALS. A year and a half after my ALS diagnosis I am, as Lou Gehrig famously said, lucky. I am alive. Of those diagnosed the same day as me, nearly one-fifth are dead. This time next year, nearly half will be dead. I am also lucky in that I can still walk, speak and hug my young daughters. And while I am lucky to be alive—as you can hear in my voice—my body is starting to fail me. Despite this, I sit here filled with hope. Why? Because we can actually cure ALS. How? By fully and boldly funding the fight against ALS. Just like you did with HIV 30 years ago. And when you do, it will help unlock cures for Alzheimer's, Parkinson's, and beyond. The research this Subcommittee has funded over the last decade enables me to say—and truly believe—that it is no longer a question of if we will find cures for ALS, but when. The opportunity to end ALS is here. Now. But to do

so requires a significant, bold new investment to make when "as soon as possible." In 2017, NIH spent approximately $13,000 on ALS research per person in the U.S. who died from ALS. We spend between 3 to 16 times that amount on diseases that kill a fraction of the people that ALS does. We spend 5 to 10 times that amount in public and private care costs for people living with ALS. Much of which is shouldered by families fighting ALS. Imagine, for a moment, if we spent the same amount on cures for ALS as we do on caring for those given this death sentence? If we did, we would finally end ALS. . . . I know you don't often hear from people with ALS in hearings like these. You don't because ALS is a relentless churn. We are diagnosed. We die. Quickly. We don't have time to advocate. Every day is a fight for survival. And it is a fight we will all lose. All of us.[1]

I must underscore two further elements of his speech in addition to its conception of the relation between science and politics: the analogy with HIV research and Brian's observation that most people diagnosed with ALS do not have time to advocate.

First of all, whether ALS will be more like HIV, as Brian suggested in 2019, in which adequate mobilization and funding led to lifesaving therapies, or if it will be more like Huntington's, in which a monogenic disorder, still after decades of intense research and funding, at times almost limitless funding, has remained ensconced in a hole in knowledge is today impossible to say.[2] Second, and this is what is important for me in this last chapter, rooted as it is in the set of exchanges that I had with Gwen, anchored in her efforts to speak out, to call for action, for herself and for others, is what Brian evoked concerning the question of time and the use of that time, a question of how someone, someone like Gwen, makes use of her time and the voice she has, to make those calls, to invoke, to advocate.

Brian's speech was given three months after I AM ALS was founded by Brian and his wife Sandra Abrevaya. Creating the organization was a response to a question Brian says he kept asking himself after his diagnosis: "Why do patients feel so disempowered in this fight?" He had been in touch with an organization called the ALS Therapy Development Institute (ALS TDI), which operates on a unique model, that rather than raising money to distribute to outside researchers, it acts as a fundraising organization that funds its own laboratory: in other words, a paradoxical entity that could be called a nonprofit biotech company. Given the existence of the ALS TDI, the financing of external researchers by other ALS organizations (notably ALSA), and that, between 2013 and 2019, the National Institutes of Health increased its investment in ALS research from

$39 million to $105 million, it was crucial to clarify the remit of any new organization in the ALS landscape: I AM ALS would raise awareness of the disease; centralize scattered resources for patients, which in turn could more easily connect them with clinical trials urgently in need of suitable subjects; and bring only new donors into the ALS fight or reengage lapsed donors, rather than cannibalizing a small pool of existing ones.

A key issue I AM ALS has worked on is engaging in serious dialogue with the FDA about how to create a regulatory environment that can adequately support ALS research. The agency has historically failed to give adequate guidance to pharmaceutical companies on drug development for ALS, and the group's pressure helped bring about the publication of a guidance document in September 2019. The main points of the nonbinding guidance were that drug companies are encouraged to discuss with patients with ALS what their expectations from an ALS drug are, which is to say, to have their input as to what a good outcome would be, meaning input from patients as to what outcomes other than a "cure" may count as worthwhile.

The guidance moreover encourages the development of new outcome measures, which is to say other than the Functional Rating Scale, whose limits have already been explored in part 2 of this book. The guidance encourages sponsors to think about drug delivery devices, especially in the case of intrathecal delivery, as well as to be wary of overly exclusionary criteria, criteria that drug sponsors may nevertheless have (some) reason to justify scientifically. The guidance indicates that while such criteria may help to show the effect of drugs, broader inclusion criteria "allow more rapid trial enrollment, potentially accelerating drug development."[3] The guidance also states that "an acceptable approach could include enrollment of a broad population with the conduct of the primary analysis in a study subset defined based on clinical characteristics and/or biomarkers, and analyses of the broader population being secondary and supportive."

On a crucial point, the FDA remained unchanged: that there must be a control group for an ALS trial given the likelihood of adverse events or death during a trial. What the FDA then means by "control group" is left somewhat underdetermined, since they recognize that "no patient should be denied effective therapies in order to be randomized to a placebo-only arm." They suggest several ways to "minimize" exposure to placebo, including the use of placebo up to a defined point of "clinically meaningful worsening in disease," after which the patient can be transferred to open-label investigational treatment. They also encourage trials to include the specification for long-term open-label extension after the completion of the randomized portion of the trial.

Possibly: February 2020

I waved to Gwen as she walked into the waiting area of the ALS clinic and introduced myself to Nathan for the first time, while Gwen went to check in with front office for her quarterly visit. She came back irritated: it had already been a hectic morning, terrible traffic, the dog, emails, no time for coffee, getting an Uber, getting downstairs, getting through the front door of their apartment building, to be on time. People have lots of different experiences of running late; less common is the experience of running late because of the mismatch between your physical capacities and the infrastructure of the world in which one lives. "Why do I have to show my ID and insurance each time I come? Unzip the purse. Fiddle to find the card. . . . It's not like going to the GP for an annual checkup. It's at least four times a year." I took the couple to their assigned room and went to tell the team that they were there.

The respiratory therapists came in, enthused to see Gwen. "I love it that you have your appointments early!" Colette said. "The morning is people at their best." Everybody laughed, but likely for different reasons. Laura listened to her breathing: "Nice deep breath. Pretty perfect." Asked if she gets headaches in the morning, Gwen replied that she has been a "clencher" all her life, so the headaches she gets are "due to the clenching; it's just me, not the ALS just me." She scored 87 on the FVC, and they spared her the inspiratory tests because she has ruptured eardrums from diving as a teenager.

Pia was next to see how Gwen was doing with speech. Fs and Vs "are hard to spit out." Gwen said she is self-conscious about it and indicated that she is tough on herself. Pia emphasized that she could hear how she is using strategies, particularly slowing down speech and overarticulating: "You are preserving clarity, which is great."

"Have you been voice banking?"

Gwen confirmed that she has, and Nathan did an exaggerated cough: no one took up his intervention, which may have been aimed at inviting Gwen to say that while it is true she had been enrolled in projects to do voice banking, the actual work of doing the recordings of speech elements, words, and phrases that she will be able to use in the future if she becomes unable to speak was something that she had not yet been able to complete, at that time, and indeed found it very difficult to bring herself to do. In the conversations she and I had had about voice banking, it was clear that talking about doing it, preparing to do it, confronted her, confronts the person who undertakes such storage, with a future that is being anticipated and for which the hope is that it can be deferred for as long as possible.

Gwen explained that she was enrolled in Google's Project Euphonia, and Pia followed up by saying that while it's great to be involved in research, it would be good to do it on a commercial platform as well, so that there is defined stability in terms of using it on everyday technology. As already developed in part 2, the team's orientation is technical, and the dynamics of psychic investment, of the emotional work of confrontation with loss, in the process of storing her voice, was not part of what could be taken up in the setting of the clinic.

So far at this clinic visit (at the end of February 2020), it is worth repeating that Gwen's breathing scores had been noted as remarkably stable since her last visit in November 2019, especially since it has been over three years since symptom onset. Second, it can be noted that a question was raised as to how to keep her still very good capacity to express herself in voice. These two points will be interconnected in what happened next during the visit with Dr. Blumen.

"I'm excited to see breathing measurements are stable. Speech stable. Swallow is okay. You'll see occupational therapy for the issues you are having with [using] the keyboard." Dr. Blumen summarized the state of affairs and then asked whether the pain Gwen had reported in November following the BrainStorm trial had cleared up. It had. The BrainStorm trial requires a lumbar puncture, which is variable in terms of physical pain postintervention. "And the Genentech study?" she asked. "Or did you decide not to do it?" Gwen did wish to do it, and she explained that it is on hold for the moment.

"Others?"

Gwen said that she would like to enroll in the "platform trial," organized by the Healey ALS Center at Massachusetts General. A platform trial is a clinical trial with a single master protocol in which multiple treatments are evaluated simultaneously and in a rolling open-ended time scale. Over time, as results come in, the trial can adapt, dropping futile treatments, declaring one or more treatments superior, or adding new treatments to be tested during the course of a trial, which is a long-term "platform" that remains open "until successful cures are found," in the words of the Healey Center. It has been set up as a perpetual multicenter, multiregimen trial evaluating the safety and efficacy of a series of investigational products for the treatment of ALS, grouped into "regimens," with each regimen made up of a different drug or drugs. Each regimen consists of a placebo-controlled trial. Participants have an equal chance to be randomized to all regimens that are active at the time of screening. Once randomized to a regimen, participants are then again randomized in a 3:1 ratio to either study drug or placebo.

"Are you eligible?" Dr. Blumen asked.

"Criteria haven't been released yet. So one of the problems is that it's three years from onset. I might not make that by sixty days."

"I have here [in the chart] that you started to fall in February 2017."

"Is there any way, if that's the only limit, is there a workaround?"

"Maybe . . . I think that would be difficult . . . the fact that you had weakness and then the fall. Are they going to get going before May?"

"They said they'd want to enroll by the end of the month. Point is: hopefully you and I can work together if I meet the rest of the criteria."

"It might not be ideal for the trial: I have November 2016 weakness started, then the fall."

"Can we update that?"

"I don't know if I'd want to update that in our system: it would mean changing all the notes going back over three years, there are notes which have gone out, for my license, it wouldn't be ethical. And then for the trials, enrolling people with longer symptom times could distort what is seen as efficacy."

Nathan intervened on this specific point, echoing the discussions within I AM ALS. "I'm in business analytics. If it's just a matter of mathematics, there should be resources made available to include as many people as possible." He described a meeting he and Gwen had been part of, with representatives from ACT UP, to discuss how patients can participate in transforming clinical trial design.

"It gets tricky," Dr. Blumen replied, "because the FDA have criteria for approval. One thing to think about is if you enroll in Platform, imagine if the stem cells are effective. You've done well, better than expected. I didn't expect you to have such good breathing results."

"Can you explain what that means?" Gwen asked.

"Once it starts to be abnormal, say 87 percent, I haven't seen it hold stable. Over 100 [percent of predicted forced vital capacity] I've seen it stay stable; once it starts to deteriorate, I've not seen it stabilize. It's possible it's the stem cells, if you got them. Let's have a look." Dr. Blumen compared the timeline of injections with breathing figures: first injection was December 17, 2018. Breathing was starting to become affected before then, 86 percent. Then from 86 to 83 percent. Then 84 percent. After all the stem cell injections 97 percent. That's interesting. Today 87 percent.

"It's hard because there is physical uncertainty in the test," Nathan said.

From Isolation to a Sense of Hope: May–November 2020

Two months into the COVID-19 pandemic and still at the front end of what people all over the world would come to call "lockdown," at the end of May, I joined Gwen and Nathan for her next clinic visit by videoconference. In-person visits were on hold. Gwen narrated that her speech continued to decline and that although the power in her legs is still good, she did have a fall earlier in the month.

It shook her up pretty bad. She has a tendency to fall backward, and this was no different. She hit her head, and her neck was pretty sore afterward. "My confidence was rattled, slowly I'm getting my confidence back. I'm still ginger when I walk, I use a walker. Tend to clutch on tightly." Nathan followed up by saying that it's hard "in a COVID world" trying to get enough physical activity. "It's a double isolation between COVID and ALS," Gwen said.

Prompted to explain what happened with the fall, Gwen described the event: picking something up off the floor. She quickly moved on to say how helpful the physical therapy program has been and that with the assistance of the physical therapist, she has been able to tailor and adapt her movements, to help get her confidence back. The team asked Gwen and Nathan how they have been coping more generally. Even though her breathing has been strong, they told the team that they have been keeping very strictly to the stay-at-home order. This in itself, Nathan said, is not what has been most difficult. Rather, their concerns were twofold: what to do in an emergency, to go to the hospital or not, and what can they hope for, in terms of research and trials given that everything seems to have slowed down in terms of enrollment, or even stopped in some cases.

Gwen took the chance to underscore that she has in effect timed out from the Healey Platform trial at Massachusetts General and made a link to the difference in efforts between a pandemic and a rare disease. "I understand that ALS is not a pandemic but in such a short period of time, there's been such a massive effort to find a solution." Nathan added that the conjuncture of the pandemic "exposes the slowness of the machine, because it's been designed to be slow. If you put the screws to people, they go faster. If you want to do something, with unlimited resources, you can do anything." Echoing Brian's testimony, and notwithstanding the countercase of Huntington's disease, there is a strong sense from those affected by this illness that more could be done if resources and effort and urgency were increased.

As time drew on, and the early dramatic stages of the pandemic waned, it slowly began to seem plausible that they could get back in motion, to orient themselves forward in time. Gwen grew up in Connecticut, where her family still lives. They were able to go for a trip to visit with Gwen's family in October 2020, which in addition to giving them time to be with each other, as a couple, was also an opportunity for Gwen to reach out to Massachusetts General, to ask if they had a place in a new clinical trial. While they didn't for that particular drug, they said that they did have space for her on the expanded access program for CNM-au8, gold nanocrystals in a drinkable solution that may help ameliorate cellular–energy deficits and oxidative stress.

Gwen was given an appointment for three weeks' time, which would have been the day before they flew back home to California. Undeterred, she asked if she could have an earlier appointment and got one in five days: "We drove up to Boston, COVID test, lab result back, and at 4 P.M. I was in clinic getting a first dose. You can do stuff if you have the knowledge, if you're in the right location, if you can self-advocate and have resources."

The week after they left, they went back to Boston for twenty-two hours, for Gwen to give blood and urine for biomarkers. Even though she is not part of the trial, they wished to collect data on it. The clinic indicated they didn't have to come back to give the samples but that they would be "good citizens" if they did it. Two additional visits were planned.

Toward the end of what had been a tumultuous year, there was a sense of positivity and of hope in what the couple were willing to share with me. "Emotionally it was really good," Nathan said of the trip to Massachusetts General. "There's energy, optimism. They think they can make a dent in this [the lack of effective therapies]." I asked whether this was contrastive with the experience in California: "It's not that they focus on the negative, it's that the [best] possible outcome is no change."

"There's always this fear that Dr. Blumen has seen something that I haven't," Gwen added. "She is cautious, less speculative. Maybe it's better."

I heard an ambivalence in the desire for hope, linked to the question of its foundation, its reality.

"Hope is all we have in this disease. It's a thing to cling to," Nathan said.

A New Phase

The company BrainStorm released their topline phase III trial data on November 17, 2020. The clinical trial data did not show statistical significance in the primary efficacy end point: a "responder analysis" evaluating the proportion of participants who experienced a 1.25 points per month improvement in the posttreatment Revised Amyotrophic Lateral Sclerosis Functional Rating Scale (ALSFRS-R) slope. It showed numerical improvement in a specific subgroup, specified *prior* to the trial (unlike for Edaravone, as explained in chapter 3), of those with 35 or more points on the functional rating scale (FRS) at baseline. Simply put, top-line data showed that 34.7 percent of patients who received the drug had a slower disease progression—as assessed with the ALSFRS-R—compared with those given a placebo, 27.7 percent. The reason this result did not achieve statistical significance is because the placebo group response exceeded those reported in other ALS trials. When comparing mean scores between placebo and the group that received the drug, no significant group differences were observed in ALSFRS-R over the seven months of treatment (–5.52 in the NurOwn group vs. −5.88 in the placebo group). Again, greater treatment responses were seen in a prespecified group of participants with less advanced disease, meaning that there were clinically significant results even if not statistically significant results.

Hence, Dr. Merit Cudkowicz, one of the principal investigators of the trial and director of the Healey Center for ALS and chair of neurology at Massachusetts General Hospital, as well as professor of neurology at Harvard University, was able to state that,

> We found a clinically meaningful response to NurOwn in a prespecified group of patients (greater than or equal to 35 ALSFRS-R at baseline). A change in pre- to post-treatment slope of 1.25 or more is substantial and clinically important. Given the heterogeneity of ALS, it is not surprising that measurement of treatment effect may be influenced by disease severity including the behavior of disease progression rates at the lower end of the scale. It is important to fully explore this finding. In addition, NurOwn was observed to have its clear intended biological effects with important changes in the pre-specified disease and drug related biomarkers.[4]

In mid-December, the company opened an Expanded Access Program, developed in partnership with the FDA, which allows clinicians to prescribe NurOwn, at no cost, to those who completed the phase III trial and who meet specific eligibility criteria, notably an FRS score of greater than 35.

On hearing this news, Gwen reached out to the site in California where she had been enrolled in the BrainStorm trial. "Out of the fifty patients enrolled at my site in BrainStorm," she told me, "they thought I would be one to benefit most from compassionate use." But there was a catch: "I was on an investigational drug at Mass Gen," the gold nanoparticles Au8. "I wanted to be transparent so I told them [the California trial site] and I asked if I could be in both. The possibility of drug interaction was an issue. They don't want data compromised by use of other drugs." Gwen asked if she could talk with Massachusetts General first and get back to her BrainStorm trial site within forty-eight hours. They agreed. She was keen not to let her place go but wanted things done properly. She spoke with the team in Boston, and they agreed that it would be best to get into the expanded access program for BrainStorm.

"So I called my trial site, and they told me they gave my slot away."

What then followed is a highly particular, although perhaps not uncommon, experience where poor organization, scientific indetermination, and the presence and absence of (minimal) consideration for people all came together.

The person who had already given her expanded access slot away advised Gwen to stay on Au8: "Stay on the other drug, the data is better," Gwen was told.

This statement, rather than being based on scientific results, was arbitrary. The person in question "has never believed in NurOwn," she told me.

Never one to be deterred, Gwen called a representative from BrainStorm. From this conversation, Gwen learned that each trial site needed to request slots for expanded access directly from the company. At her site, initially zero slots were requested. Gwen narrated to me the conversation that the BrainStorm representative said she had with a trial site representative: "You gotta have at least one patient interested in it?!!" Finally, the site acquiesced and asked for a single slot, which is what was given away. Either another slot would have to be advocated for, or another participating site would have to be asked to transfer one of their slots.

Testament to Gwen's refusal to give up on her desire, a few days later, she received a call from the representative, with a hopeful but vague enunciation to the effect of "we might have good news." She found her place.

THE INCURABLE AND THE POSSIBLE

Why conduct an inquiry into knowing, caring for, and giving form to life with ALS? To not have done it would have been, in my case, a way of avoiding something that had the mark of necessity, given the prior work I had done with people who had sought to voluntarily end their lives when faced with a suffering that they no longer wished to countenance: a necessity of investigating possibilities, other ways of confronting, of facing the incurable.

The incurable is not equivalent to death and can be constituted in a "nonrapport" with death, which is another way of saying that this nonrapport is a way of bracketing human beings' structural relation with finitude, so as to not treat the one who suffers from the illness as already dead. There is a certitude about the incurability of this illness that stems from our ignorance, a lack in our (medical) knowledge that also provides the indetermination about what, in fact, it is: what will happen, how it will unfold.

Dr. Blumen, despite her vast experience, in which the outcome is in effect, at least from one point of view, the same, always insisted on the particularity of each person's trajectory and the fact that one really does never know how it will unfold. That this illness has a defined and definite set of characteristics, while necessary, is to a degree beside the point, when what counts, one by one, is how the person has it. This, for me, is the lesson of these clinics and what can be taken, in terms of knowledge, from what I was able to learn from Frances, Emma, and Gwen: what will you do and express with the body, the speaking body you have, in the time that remains? This is a lesson that I, for one, have endeavored to grasp and to carry forward in writing this book.

Is it only chance that the three narratives all came from women? I didn't choose them. Gwen and Emma responded to my desire to know something about a life when a body is subject to this illness: they were willing to talk. With respect to Frances, I was taken, enamored is the right word, with her writing, not only her reflections, which were considered, but also the very act of making every letter count, given her impossibility of speaking.

Necessarily, the question of sense was posed: I'm supposed to learn something, Emma said, which I heard as the high bar of me having to make knowledge with this encounter, while she asked for her blessing.

The question of sense was also, in my discussions with Gwen, posed but not concerning the illness itself: never was there the question of a meaning to be given to the illness. Sense was given instead to the call for action, the call for more experiments, more trials, more effort, to not or to never equate, or mistake, the incurable for the not possible. The universal of this illness is nevertheless not-all. Not-all of the one subject to ALS is subject to this universal.

When Gwen first spoke to me about The Shrug, I was concerned. The gesture, in her telling, or rather, in my reception of her telling of it, was indexed to what I had taken to be an impossibility. One hundred fifty years of knowledge, and yet still this illness is incurable. The absence of a cure, or any significant treatment, is a contingent one, not a logical impossibility. It is located in the temporal register of "for now." My concern was to have confused the registers, that I had succumbed to The Shrug, to its silence, and in so doing, and this was my worry, that I had given it a meaning as something more than contingent, a sense that it pointed to a necessary impossibility.

Let's try another reading then of The Shrug: as a sign of a failure that is contingent, a lack, an inability to respond in the present to a demand for treatment, for a cure, this gesture, this *mute* sign, this hole in knowledge, asks of the person who receives it to compose with this lack in knowledge about something whose existence is undeniable: a body that is suffering.

The Shrug would then be something other than a sign of the universal fatality of this illness: it is the sign of an absence in which that universality does not cover over everything, leaving space for the question of a desire that can persist, that can be given a form, aside from any demand: demand for cure, certainly, but also, as we saw with Mrs. Liu and Emma, demand for death because of the absence of cure. In the three narratives that make up the last part of the book, there are three singular ways of responding to such lack: for each person, their work, their words won't cure their bodies but can give a form to their wish to know something and do something *with*, *in spite of*, and *because of* that lack: the epistle, the plea, the call to action.

The stories of these three women and the case of this particular illness thus open onto the broader theme of how people orient themselves by way of "spaces of experience" and "horizons of expectation," to use Reinhart Koselleck's terms. To the degree that incurability is a contingent historical phenomenon and not a logical necessity, following Koselleck, such contingency is conceivable only through this pair of concepts, experience and expectation.

There is a universal aspect to the articulation of experience and expectation in the case of ALS, which is that this incurability, rooted in a combination of certitude and indetermination, is identical for all. There is a local or an institutional aspect, which I have taken up not at the level of a culture, "the US," but at the level of how different medical-clinical practices orient themselves to evaluative and normative statements about life with this illness, based on their clinical experience and clinical expectations, what these clinics seek to make present, in the present. There is finally the level at which an individual living with the illness articulates experience and expectation, which I have already indicated with the questions, what can I know and what should I do, to which Kant's third critical question should be added: what may I hope for? The universal is not-all. Koselleck, with his characteristic clarity, writes, "Whoever believes himself capable of deducing his expectations in their entirety from his experience is in error. If something happens in a way different from what was expected, one learns from it. On the other hand, whoever fails to base his expectations on experience is likewise in error. He should have known better. There is clearly an aporia here that is resolved in the course of time."[1]

Emma said she was supposed to learn something from her experience. What appeared for her, what she was able to name and to say, was to have learned something about her demand (for the grace of God) that went beyond her demand for death. For Gwen, after her breathing scores dipped, following participation in the BrainStorm trial, they went up and stabilized. Something will be learned either way when she finds out if she was on placebo or therapy. And moreover, her horizon of expectation will keep reaching beyond whatever may result from any given trial. The call to action continues. Frances, for her part, learned to welcome the surprise and the use she could make of a body that exists, that insists, in spite of all. As Koselleck puts it, regarding prognosis, "Diagnosis has precedence and is made on the basis of the data of experience. Seen in this way, the space of experience, open toward the future, draws the horizon of expectation out of itself. Experiences release and direct prognoses. But prognoses are also defined by the requirement that they expect something. Concern related to the broader or narrower field of action produces expectations into which fear and hope also enter. Alternative conditions must be taken into consideration; possibilities come into play that always contain more than can be realized in the coming reality."[2] Haud Guéguen and Laurent Jeanpierre name this capacity for expectation to exceed the space of experience as the "perspective of the possible." The possible, in their view, is a critical operator on the given contours of a reality; it is an operator of experimentation and a "defiance with respect to the existent."[3] At the same time, the very nature of that existent requires interrogation, and following Koselleck, such defiance is rooted in such existence and must take account of it.

To return to our maxim, in the purely formal injunction from the ALS clinic, to live as well as possible as long as possible, the possible is facilitated by the experimental character of a desire that is both supported by and yet moves beyond any particular demand (to go on mechanical ventilation or not, to ask for a feeding tube or not, to request lethal medication to end your own life or not). The possible is constrained, moreover, by way of what is happening in a body, its sheer existence, which is simultaneously the case and impossible to grasp in and of itself (prediscursively), an existence that is approached in the identification of words through which to orient that search for the possible. As Gwen put it, of the moment before arriving at the diagnosis, if only my body could speak. And she did. The possible, the experimentation with a form for life, is tied to the existent, what is happening in a body, but how it is tied is precisely the open question, for each, one by one.

Notes

PREFACE

1. VITALMORTEL. My thanks to the French Agence Nationale de la Recherche (ANR-17-CE36-0007).

2. Janine Barbot and Nicolas Dodier, "Victims and the Ecologies of Reparation Dispositifs in the Contaminated Growth Hormone Case: Comparative Perspectives on Recovery after a Health Disaster," in *Rethinking Post-Disaster Recovery*, ed. Laura Centemeri, Sezin Topçu, J. Peter Burgess (London: Routledge, 2021).

3. Frances McGill, *Go Not Gently: Letters from a Patient with Amyotrophic Lateral Sclerosis* (New York: Arno Press, 1980), 59–60.

4. Kenneth Burke, "Literature as Equipment for Living," in *The Philosophy of Literary Form* (Berkeley: University of California Press, 1973).

5. Key examples include but are not limited to the different ways that both Bourdieu and Foucault took up the Stoics: Pierre Bourdieu, *Practical Reason: On the Theory of Action*, trans. Randal Johnson and Others (Stanford, CA: Stanford University Press, 1998 [1994]), 77; Michel Foucault, *The Hermeneutics of the Subject: Lectures at the Collège de France, 1981–1982*, ed. Frédéric Gros, trans. Graham Burchell (New York: Palgrave Macmillan, 2005 [2001]), 308. Michael Pollack took up Bourdieu's theory of the habitus to consider how individuals pragmatically faced and navigated Nazi concentration camps: Michael Pollak, *L'expérience concentrationnaire: Essai sur le maintien de l'identité sociale* (Paris: Métailié, 1990).

INTRODUCTION

1. Jeannette Pols and Sarah Limburg, "A Matter of Taste? Quality of Life in Day-to-Day Living with ALS and a Feeding Tube," *Culture, Medicine, and Psychiatry* 40, no. 3 (2016): 361–382.

2. Dikaios Sakellariou, "Enacting Varieties of Subjectivity through Practices of Care: A Story of Living with Motor Neuron Disease," *Qualitative Health Research* 26, no. 14 (2016): 1902–1910; Dikaios Sakellariou, Gail Boniface, and Paul Brown, "Using Joint Interviews in a Narrative-Based Study on Illness Experiences," *Qualitative Health Research* 23, no. 11 (2013): 1563–1570; Dikaios Sakellariou, "Home Modifications and Ways of Living Well," *Medical Anthropology* 34, no. 5 (2015): 456–469; Narelle Warren and Dikaios Sakellariou, "Neurodegeneration and the Intersubjectivities of Care," *Medical Anthropology* 39 (2020): 1–15.

3. Chelsey R. Carter, "The 'Truth' about ALS: Reconciling Bias, Motives, and Etiological Gaps," *Somatosphere*, http://somatosphere.net/2020/als-bias-motives-etiological-gaps.html/. See also Chelsea R. Carter, "Gaslighting: ALS, Anti-Blackness, and Medicine," *Feminist Anthropology* 3 (2022): 235–245.

4. Vololona Rabeharisoa and Michel Callon, "L'implication des malades dans les activités de recherche soutenues par l'Association française contre les myopathies," *Sciences sociales et santé* 16, no. 3 (1998): 41–65.

5. Vololona Rabeharisoa and Michel Callon, "The Growing Engagement of Emergent Concerned Groups in Political and Economic Life: Lessons from the French Association

of Neuromuscular Disease Patients," *Science, Technology, & Human Values* 33, no. 2 (2008): 241.

6. Michel Callon, "An Essay on Framing and Overflowing: Economic Externalities Revisited by Sociology" *Sociological Review* 46, no. 1 (1998): 244–269.

7. Alice Rivière, *The Dingdingdong Manifesto*, in Katrin Solhdju, *Testing Knowledge: Toward an Ecology of Diagnosis, Preceded by the Dingdingdong Manifesto*, trans. Damien Bright (Goleta, CA: 3Ecologies Books, Punctum Books, 2021), 41.

8. Narelle Warren and D. Ayton, "(Re) Negotiating Normal Every Day: Phenomeno-logical Uncertainty in Parkinson's Disease," in *Disability, Normalcy, and the Everyday*, ed. Gareth M. Thomas and Dikaios Sakellariou (London: Routledge, 2018), 142.

9. Hans-Jörg Rheinberger, *On Historicizing Epistemology: An Essay* (Stanford, CA: Stanford University Press, 2010).

10. Bharat Venkat, *At the Limits of Cure* (Durham, NC: Duke University Press, 2021).

11. Jonathan Darrow, Ameet Sarpatwari, Jerry Avorn, and Aaron S. Kesselheim, "Practical, Legal, and Ethical Issues in Expanded Access to Investigational Drugs," *New England Journal of Medicine* 372 (2015): 279–286.

PART 1. KNOWLEDGE

1. Erwin H. Ackerknecht, "Elisha Bartlett and the Philosophy of the Paris Clinical School," *Bulletin of the History of Medicine* 24, no. 1 (1950): 43–60; Toby Gelfand, "Gestation of the Clinic," Medical History 25, no. 2 (1981): 169–180, https://doi.org/10.1017/S0025727300034360.

2. Michel Foucault, *The Birth of the Clinic: An Archaeology of Medical Perception* (London: Routledge [1976], Taylor & Francis e-Library, 2003), x–xi.

3. Flurin Condrau, "The Patient's View Meets the Clinical Gaze," *Social History of Medicine* 20, no. 3 (2007): 525–540; Roy Porter, "The Patient's View: Doing Medical History from Below," *Theory and Society* 14 (1985): 175–198; David Armstrong, "The Patient's View," *Social Science and Medicine* 18 (1984): 737–744.

4. The roots of the anatomo-clinical method are frequently identified in the work of Giovanni Battista Morgagni, an Italian anatomist, and his *De Sedibus et causis morborum per anatomem indagatis* [*Of the seats and causes of diseases investigated through anatomy*] (Venetiis: Remondini, 1761).

1. THE EMERGENCE OF A DIAGNOSTIC CERTITUDE

1. Charles Bell, *The Nervous System of the Human Body: Embracing the Papers Delivered to the Bengal Society on the Subject of the Nerves. With Appendix, Containing Cases and Letters of Consultation on Nervous Diseases* (London: Longmans & Co, 1836), 248.

2. Bell, *The Nervous System of the Human Body*, 248.

3. Sir Charles Bell, *Letters of Sir Charles Bell, K.H., F.R.S.L. & E.: Selected from His Correspondence with His Brother George Joseph Bell* (London: J. Murray, 1870), 170–171.

4. Carin Berkowitz, *Charles Bell and the Anatomy of Reform* (Chicago: University of Chicago Press, 2015).

5. Jean-Martin Charcot, *Charcot, the Clinician: The Tuesday Lessons: Excerpts from Nine Case Presentations on General Neurology Delivered at the Salpêtrière Hospital in 1887–88*, trans. with commentary by Christopher G. Goetz (New York: Raven Press, 1987).

6. The spectacle of Charcot's work at the Pitié-Salpêtrière, as well as the crucial interconnection of the image-spectacle, techniques of photography, and Charcot's rediscovery of the category of hysteria, has been shown in George Didi-Huberman's classic study, *Invention of Hysteria: Charcot and the Photographic Iconography of the Salpêtrière* (Cambridge, MA: MIT Press, 2003).

7. Charcot, *Charcot, the Clinician*.

8. Guillaume Duchenne de Boulogne, "Paralysie musculaire progressive de la langue, du voile du palais et des lèvres; affection non encore décrite comme espèce morbide distincte," *Archives générales de médecine* 16 (1860): 283–296.

9. Charcot, *Charcot, the Clinician*, 170.

10. People with Broca's aphasia (nonfluent/expressive) have trouble speaking fluently, but their comprehension can be relatively preserved. Broca's aphasia results from injury to speech and language brain areas such the left hemisphere inferior frontal gyrus, among others. Such damage is often a result of stroke but may also occur due to brain trauma. As in other types of aphasia, intellectual and cognitive capabilities not related to speech and language may be fully preserved.

11. Charcot, *Charcot, the Clinician*, 174.

12. A co-occurrence that I revisit in chapter 2.

13. Charcot, *Charcot, the Clinician*, 173.

14. Sanger Brown, "The Neuron in Medicine," *Journal of the American Medical Association* 26 (1896): 10.

15. W. R. Gowers, *A Manual of Diseases of the Nervous System*, 3rd ed., vol. 1 (London: J. & A. Churchill), 214–215.

16. Neurologist and Charcot specialist Christopher Goetz wrote of the Charcot–Gowers dispute that Charcot believed that the amyotrophy was, in fact, due to spread of the disease from the lateral columns to the spinal and bulbar gray matter. This hypothesis unleashed a debate between Charcot and Gowers, who contested that the degeneration was a uniform and single event. He opposed Charcot's term "amyotrophic lateral sclerosis," because it implied that the primary lesion was in the lateral columns, with the atrophy a secondary phenomenon, which he disagreed with. Christopher Goetz, "Amyotrophic Lateral Sclerosis: Early Contributions of Jean-Martin Charcot," *Muscle & Nerve* 23, no. 3 (2000): 336–343.

17. François Amilcar Aran, "Recherches sur une maladie non encore décrite du système musculaire (atrophie musculaire progressive)," *Archives générales de médecine* 14 (1850): 172–214.

18. Lawrence C. McHenry and Fielding Hudson Garrison, *Garrison's History of Neurology* (Springfield, IL: Thomas, 1969), 279.

19. McHenry and Garrison, *Garrison's History of Neurology*, 437; Jules Bernard Luys, "Atrophie Musculaire Progressive: Lésions Histologiques De La Substance Grise de la Moelle Epinière," *Gazette médicale de Paris* 3, no. 15 (1860): 505.

20. Michel Foucault, *The Birth of the Clinic: An Archaeology of Medical Perception* (London: Taylor & Francis e-Library, 2003), 131.

21. Foucault, *The Birth of the Clinic*, 122.

22. Foucault, *The Birth of the Clinic*, 134.

23. Christopher G. G. Goetz, "Jean-Martin Charcot and the Anatomo-Clinical Method of Neurology," in *Handbook of Clinical Neurology: History of Neurology*, ed. Stanley Finger, Francois Boller, and Kenneth L. Tyler (Cambridge, MA: Elsevier, 2009), 207.

24. Goetz, "Jean-Martin Charcot and the Anatomo-Clinical Method of Neurology," 208.

25. Wilhelm Heinrich Erb, "Über einen wenig bekannten Spinalen Symptomencomplex," *Berliner klinische Wochenschrift* 12 (1875): 357–359.

26. Goetz, "Jean-Martin Charcot and the Anatomo-Clinical Method of Neurology," 209.

27. Goetz, "Jean-Martin Charcot and the Anatomo-Clinical Method of Neurology."

28. Martin R. Turner, Michael Swash, and George C. Ebers, "Lockhart Clarke's Contribution to the Description of Amyotrophic Lateral Sclerosis," *Brain: A Journal of Neurology* 133, no. 11 (2010): 3470–3479.

29. Turner, Swash, and Ebers, "Lockhart Clarke's Contribution to the Description of Amyotrophic Lateral Sclerosis."

30. Turner, Swash, and Ebers, "Lockhart Clarke's Contribution to the Description of Amyotrophic Lateral Sclerosis," my emphasis.

31. Foucault, *The Birth of the Clinic*, 134.

32. Turner, Swash, and Ebers, "Lockhart Clarke's Contribution to the Description of Amyotrophic Lateral Sclerosis," 3474.

33. Lockhart Clarke, "Morbid Anatomy of the Nervous Centres," *Edinburgh Medical Journal* 8 (1862): 177.

34. Clarke, "Morbid Anatomy of the Nervous Centres."

35. Foucault, *The Birth of the Clinic*, 137.

36. Gowers, *Manual*, 494.

37. Gowers, *Manual*.

38. Gowers, *Manual*.

39. Martin R. Turner and Michael Swash, "The Expanding Syndrome of Amyotrophic Lateral Sclerosis: A Clinical and Molecular Odyssey," *Journal of Neurology, Neurosurgery, and Psychiatry* 86 (2015): 668.

40. Russell Brain, *Diseases of the Nervous System*, 8th ed. (Oxford: Oxford University Press, 1969), 683.

2. NOSOLOGICAL INDETERMINATIONS

1. Pierre Marie, *Lectures on Diseases of the Spinal Cord*, trans. Montagu Lubbock (London: The New Sydenham Society, 1895 [1892]), 771.

2. D. Neary, J. S. Snowden, D. M. Mann, B. Northen, P. J. Goulding, and N. Macdermott, "Frontal Lobe Dementia and Motor Neuron Disease," *Journal of Neurology, Neurosurgery & Psychiatry* 53, no. 1 (1990): 31.

3. Neary et al., "Frontal Lobe Dementia and Motor Neuron Disease."

4. Verena Keck, *The Search for a Cause: An Anthropological Perspective on a Neurological Disease in Guam, Western Pacific* (Guam: Richard Taitano Micronesian Area Resource Center, University of Guam, 2011).

5. Motor issues are necessarily taken into account for FTD variants such as primary progressive aphasia. My thanks to Laurence Tessier for clarifying this point.

6. Marius Bordes, "Considérations sur les troubles psychiques dans le tabes, dans la sclérose en plaques et dans la sclérose latérale amyotrophique," PhD diss., Université de Toulouse, 1908.

7. Marie, quoted in Bordes, "Considérations," 54.

8. Bordes, "Considérations," 55–56.

9. William Richard Gowers, *A Manual of Diseases of the Nervous System*, 3rd ed. (Philadelphia: P. Blakiston's Son & Co., 1899), 240.

10. Bordes, "Considérations," 61.

11. Bordes, "Considérations," 63–64.

12. Bordes, "Considérations," 93.

13. Bordes, "Considérations," 96.

14. Lloyd H. Ziegler, "Psychotic and Emotional Phenomena Associated with Amyotrophic Lateral Sclerosis," *Archives of Neurology and Psychiatry* 24, no. 5 (1930): 931.

15. H. Oppenheim and E. Siemerling, "Mitteilungen über Pseudobulbärparalyse und akute Bulbärparalyse," *Berliner Klinische Wochenschrift* 46 (1886): 791–794.

16. Ziegler, "Psychotic and Emotional Phenomena Associated with Amyotrophic Lateral Sclerosis," 930.

17. Ziegler, "Psychotic and Emotional Phenomena Associated with Amyotrophic Lateral Sclerosis," 931.

18. Ziegler, "Psychotic and Emotional Phenomena Associated with Amyotrophic Lateral Sclerosis," 930.

19. Ziegler, "Psychotic and Emotional Phenomena Associated with Amyotrophic Lateral Sclerosis."

20. J. S. Wechsler and C. Davison, "Amyotrophic Lateral Sclerosis with Mental Symptoms," *Archives of Neurology and Psychiatry* xxvii (1932): 859–880.

21. Wechsler and Davison, "Amyotrophic Lateral Sclerosis with Mental Symptoms."

22. William Pryse-Phillips, *Companion to Clinical Neurology* (Oxford: Oxford University Press, 2009), 372.

23. S. Brion, A. Psimaras, J. F. Chevalier, J. Plas, G Massé, and O. Jatteau, "L'association maladie de Pick et sclerose laterale amyotrophique: Etude d'un cas anatomo-clinique et revue de la littérature," *L'Encéphale* 6 (1980): 270.

24. Jamie Talan, "Researchers Focus on Cluster of ALS Cases in Guam," *LA Times*, December 27, 1992. Cf. H. Zimmerman, *Progress Report of Work in the Laboratory of Pathology during May, 1945* (Washington, DC: US Naval Medical Research Unit Number 2, 1945).

25. Arthur Arnold, Donald Edgren, and Vincent Palladino, "ALS: Fifty Cases Observed on Guam," *Journal of Nervous and Mental Disease* 117, no. 2 (1953): 135–139.

26. Leonard T. Kurland and Donald W. Mulder, "Epidemiologic Investigations of Amyotrophic Lateral Sclerosis. Familial Aggregations Indicative of Dominant Inheritance Part I," *Neurology* 5, no. 3 (1955): 182.

27. Donald W. Mulder, Leonard Kurland, and Lorenzo L. Iriarte, "Neurologic Diseases on the Island of Guam," *U.S. Forces Medical Journal* 5 (1954): 1724–1739.

28. Mulder, Kurland, and Iriarte, "Neurologic Diseases on the Island of Guam," 1734.

29. Asao Hirano, Leonard T. Kurland, Robert S. Krooth, and Simmons Lessell, "Parkinsonism-Dementia Complex, an Endemic Disease on the Island of Guam: I. Clinical Features," *Brain* 84, no. 4 (1961): 642–643.

30. Hirano et al., "Parkinsonism-Dementia Complex," 652.

31. J. C. Steele, "Parkinsonism-Dementia Complex of Guam," *Movement Disorders* 20, suppl. 12 (2005): S99–S107.

32. Oliver Sacks, *The Island of the Color-Blind and Cycad Island* (New York: Picador, 1997), 111.

33. Suzee E. Lee, "Guam Dementia Syndrome Revisited in 2011," *Current Opinion in Neurology* 24, no. 6 (2011): 518.

34. Sacks, *The Island of the Color-Blind*, 98.

35. Sacks, *The Island of the Color-Blind*.

36. Sacks, *The Island of the Color-Blind*.

37. M. Bonduelle, P. Bouygues, R. Escourolle, and G. Lormeau, "Evolution Simultan6e d'une Sclérose Latérale Amyotrophique, d'un Syndrome Parkinsonien et d'une Démence Progressive A Propos de Deux Observations Anatomo-Cliniques Essai d'Interprétation," *Journal of the Neurological Sciences* 6 (1968): 330.

38. Nicholas Olney, Salvatore Spina, and Bruce L. Miller, "Frontotemporal Dementia," *Neurologic Clinics* 35, no. 2 (2017): 339–374.

39. S. Brion, A. Psimaras, J. F. Chevalier, J. Plas, G. Massé, and O. Jatteau, "L'association maladie de Pick et sclérose latérale amyotrophique. Etude d'un cas anatomo-clinique et revue de la littérature," *Encéphale* 6, no. 3 (1980): 259–286.

40. Brion et al., "L'association maladie de Pick," 259.

41. Brion et al., "L'association maladie de Pick."

42. Laurence Tessier, "Social Brains: On Two Neuroscientific Conceptions of Human Sociality," *BioSocieties* 14 (2019): 67–93.

43. Brion et al., "L'association maladie de Pick," 278.

44. Brion et al., "L'association maladie de Pick."

45. D. Neary, J. S. Snowden, D. M. Mann, B. Northen, P. J. Goulding, and N. Macdermott, "Frontal Lobe Dementia and Motor Neuron Disease," *Journal of Neurology, Neurosurgery & Psychiatry* 53, no. 1 (1990): 30.

46. Catherine Lomen-Hoerth, Thomas Anderson, and Bruce Miller, "The Overlap of Amyotrophic Lateral Sclerosis and Frontotemporal Dementia," *Neurology* 59, no. 7 (2002): 1078.

47. Catherine Lomen-Hoerth, J. Murphy, S. Langmore, J. H. Kramer, R. K. Olney, and B. Miller, "Are Amyotrophic Lateral Sclerosis Patients Cognitively Normal?" *Neurology* 60, no. 7 (2003): 1094.

48. Catherine Lomen-Hoerth, "Clinical Phenomenology and Neuroimaging Correlates in ALS-FTD," *Journal of Molecular Neuroscience* 45, no. 3 (2011): 656.

49. Ian R. A. Mackenzie and Howard H. Feldman, "Ubiquitin Immunohistochemistry Suggests Classic Motor Neuron Disease, Motor Neuron Disease with Dementia, and Frontotemporal Dementia of the Motor Neuron Disease Type Represent a Clinicopathologic Spectrum," *Journal of Neuropathology & Experimental Neurology* 64, no. 8 (2005): 730–739.

50. Tetsuaki Arai, Masato Hasegawa, Haruhiko Akiyama, Kenji Ikeda, Takashi Nonaka, Hiroshi Mori, David Mann, et al., "TDP-43 Is a Component of Ubiquitin-Positive Tau-Negative Inclusions in Frontotemporal Lobar Degeneration and Amyotrophic Lateral Sclerosis," *Biochemical and Biophysical Research Communications* 351, no. 3 (2006): 602–611.

51. Martin R. Turner and Michael Swash, "The Expanding Syndrome of Amyotrophic Lateral Sclerosis: A Clinical and Molecular Odyssey," *Journal of Neurology, Neurosurgery, and Psychiatry* 86, no. 6 (2015): 670.

52. Turner and Swash, "The Expanding Syndrome of Amyotrophic Lateral Sclerosis," 670. Cf. Thomas H. Bak and Siddharthan Chandran, "What Wires Together Dies Together: Verbs, Actions and Neurodegeneration in Motor Neuron Disease," *Cortex* 48, no. 7 (2012): 936–944.

53. Bak and Chandran, "What Wires Together Dies Together," 936.

54. Stefanos Geroulanos and Todd Meyers, *The Human Body in the Age of Catastrophe* (Chicago: University of Chicago Press, 2018).

55. For a person to have "a bit of a stare" is the basis of one of the diagnoses described by Laurence Tessier in her terrific article "A Flavor of Alzheimer's," *Journal of the Royal Anthropological Institute* 23, no. 2 (2017): 249–266.

PART 2. CARE

1. W. Eugene Smith, "A Country Doctor," *Life Magazine*, 1948. Cf. Ben Cosgrove, "Country Doctor: W. Eugene Smith's Landmark Photo Essay," *Life Magazine*, https://www.life.com/history/w-eugene-smiths-landmark-photo-essay-country-doctor/.

2. Antoine Sénanque, *Blouse* (Paris: Grasset, 2006). My translation.

3. Sénanque, *Blouse*.

4. R. G. Miller et al., "Practice Parameter Update: The Care of the Patient with Amyotrophic Lateral Sclerosis: Multidisciplinary Care, Symptom Management, and Cognitive/Behavioral Impairment (an Evidence-Based Review): Report of the Quality Standards Subcommittee of the American Academy of Neurology," *Neurology* 73, no. 15 (2009): 1228–1229.

5. Miller et al., "Practice Parameter Update," 1229.

3. MULTIDISCIPLINARY ALS CARE

1. Importantly, George Weisz has shown how the concept of "chronic disease" was largely an American policy construct from the first half of the twentieth century: George Weisz, *Chronic Disease in the Twentieth Century: A History* (Baltimore: JHU Press, 2014). His book underscores that it was in the 1960s and 1970s that theory transitioned into practice.

2. David Clark, *Cicely Saunders: Founder of the Hospice Movement: Selected Letters 1959–1999* (Oxford: Oxford University Press, 2005).

3. Elisabeth Kübler-Ross, *On Death and Dying* (New York: Macmillan, 1969); Roy Branson, "Is Acceptance a Denial of Death? Another Look at Kübler-Ross," *Christian Century* 92, no. 17 (1975): 46.

4. Barney Glaser and Anselm Leonard Strauss, *Awareness of Dying* (Chicago: Aldine Press, 1965).

5. Albert R. Jonsen, "Dying Right in California—The Natural Death Act," *Clinical Toxicology* 13, no. 4. (1978): 513–522; EU Parliament, Resolution 613 (1976): "Rights of the Sick and Dying."

6. Nick Kemp, *Merciful Release: The History of the British Euthanasia Movement* (Manchester: Manchester University Press, 2002).

7. Balfour M. Mount, "The Problem of Caring for the Dying in a General Hospital: The Palliative Care Unit as a Possible Solution," *Canadian Medical Association Journal* 115, no. 2 (1976): 119.

8. Michel Castra, *Bien Mourir: Sociologie des soins palliatifs* (Paris: PUF, 2003).

9. Judith Richman and Patricia Casey, "Multidisciplinary Approach to Management and Support of Patients," in *Motor Neuron Disease*, ed. Ralph W. Kuncl (London: W. B. Saunders, 2002).

10. Michel Foucault, "Polemics, Politics and Problematizations," in *Essential Works of Michel Foucault, vol. 1, Ethics: Subjectivity and Truth*, ed. Paul Rabinow, 281–301 (New York: The New Press [1984] 1997).

11. Michael Stolberg, *A History of Palliative Care, 1500–1970*, vol. 123, Philosophy and Medicine (Cham: Springer International Publishing, 2017), 151.

12. Stolberg, *A History of Palliative Care*, 158.

13. P. G. Newrick and R. Langton-Hewer, "Motor Neurone Disease: Can We Do Better? A Study of 42 Patients," *British Medical Journal (Clinical Research Ed.)* 289, no. 6444 (1984): 541.

14. Newrick and R. Langton-Hewer, "Motor Neurone Disease," 541.

15. Richard A. Smith and Forbes H. Norris, "Symptomatic Care of Patients with Amyotrophic Lateral Sclerosis," *JAMA* 234, no. 7 (1975): 715.

16. D. W. Janiszewski, J. T. Caroscio, and L. H. Wisham, "Amyotrophic Lateral Sclerosis: A Comprehensive Rehabilitation Approach," *Archives of Physical Medicine and Rehabilitation* 64, no. 7 (1983): 304–307.

17. Janiszewski, Caroscio, and Wisham, "Amyotrophic Lateral Sclerosis," 304.

18. Janiszewski, Caroscio, and Wisham, "Amyotrophic Lateral Sclerosis," 305.

19. Forbes H. Norris, Richard A. Smith, and E. H. Denys, "Motor Neurone Disease: Towards Better Care," *British Medical Journal (Clinical Research Ed.)* 291, no. 6490 (1985): 259.

20. Norris, Smith, and Denys, "Motor Neurone Disease," 262.

21. As the French sociologists Nicolas Dodier and Janine Barbot have written, regarding apparatuses, *dispositifs* in French, "The internal heterogeneity of dispositifs . . . is a crucial property that merits specific attention, both in terms of the meaning assigned to this multiplicity and its implications for studying the interactions between human

beings and dispositifs. Three other properties are also important to the conceptual appeal of dispositifs: their twofold relationship to ideals, the fact that they fulfill purposes, and their capacity to transform individuals who come into contact with them." Nicolas Dodier and Janine Barbot, "La force des dispositifs," *Annales: Histoire, Sciences Sociales* 71, no. 2 (2016): 421.

22. V. Appel, S. Stewart, G. Smith, and S. H. Appel, "A Rating Scale for Amyotrophic Lateral Sclerosis: Description and Preliminary Experience," *Annals of Neurology* 22, no. 3 (1987): 328.

23. Appel et al., "A Rating Scale for Amyotrophic Lateral Sclerosis," 328.

24. Franco Franchignoni, Gabriele Mora, Andrea Giordano, Paolo Volanti, and Adriano Chiò, "Evidence of Multidimensionality in the ALSFRS-R Scale: A Critical Appraisal on its Measurement Properties Using Rasch Analysis," *Journal of Neurology, Neurosurgery & Psychiatry* 84, no. 12 (2013): 1340–1345.

25. Michael Swash, "New Ideas on the ALS Functional Rating Scale," *Journal of Neurology, Neurosurgery & Psychiatry* 88 (2017): 371–372.

26. Swash, "New Ideas on the ALS Functional Rating Scale."

27. Andrew Eisen, "Motor Neurone Disease," in *Landmark Papers in Neurology*, ed. Martin Turner and Matthew C. Kiernan (Oxford: Oxford University Press, 2015), 257.

28. Martin R. Turner, A. Al-Chalabi, C. E. Shaw, et al., "Riluzole and Motor Neurone Disease," *Practical Neurology* 3 (2003):164.

29. Turner et al., "Riluzole and Motor Neurone Disease," 164.

30. Koji Abe, Y. Itoyama, G. Sobue, et al., "Confirmatory Double-Blind, Parallel-Group, Placebo-Controlled Study of Efficacy and Safety of Edaravone (MCI-186) in Amyotrophic Lateral Sclerosis Patients," *Amyotrophic Lateral Sclerosis and Frontotemporal Degeneration* 7–8 (2014): 610–617.

31. Masahiko Tanaka, Sakata Takeshi, Joseph Palumbo, and Makoto Akimoto, "A 24-Week, Phase III, Double-Blind, Parallel-Group Study of Edaravone (MCI-186) for Treatment of Amyotrophic Lateral Sclerosis (ALS)," *Neurology* 86, no. 16 (2016): P3, 189.

32. Tanaka et al., "A 24-Week, Phase III, Double-Blind, Parallel-Group Study of Edaravone," 189.

33. Ammar Al-Chalabi, Peter M. Andersen, Siddharthan Chandran, et al., "July 2017 ENCALS Statement on Edaravone," *Amyotrophic Lateral Sclerosis and Frontotemporal Degeneration* 18, nos. 7–8 (2017): 473.

34. Carlayne Jackson, Terry Heiman-Patterson, Pamela Kittrell, Tatyana Baranovsky, Glenn McAnanama, Laura Bower, Wendy Agnese, and Mike Martin, "Radicava (Edaravone) for Amyotrophic Lateral Sclerosis: US Experience at 1 Year after Launch," *Amyotrophic Lateral Sclerosis and Frontotemporal Degeneration* 20, nos. 7–8 (2019): 606.

35. Pam Belluck, "2 College Students Dreamed Up an A.L.S. Treatment. The Results Are In," *New York Times*, September 2, 2020.

36. Richard S. Bedlack, Timothy Vaughan, Paul Wicks, et al., "How Common Are ALS Plateaus and Reversals?" *Neurology* 86, no. 9 (2016): 808–812.

37. Vincenzo Silani, Edward J. Kasarskis, and Nobuo Yanagisawa, "Nutritional Management in Amyotrophic Lateral Sclerosis: A Worldwide Perspective," *Journal of Neurology* 245, no. 2 (1998): S13–S19.

38. Silani, Kasarskis, and Yanagisawa, "Nutritional Management in Amyotrophic Lateral Sclerosis," S14.

39. Richard A. Smith and Forbes H. Norris, "Symptomatic Care of Patients with Amyotrophic Lateral Sclerosis," *Journal of the American Medical Association* 234, no. 7 (1975): 716.

40. Smith and Norris, "Symptomatic Care of Patients with Amyotrophic Lateral Sclerosis," 716.

41. P. G. Newrick and R. Langton-Hewer, "Motor Neurone Disease: Can We Do Better? A Study of 42 Patients," *British Medical Journal (Clinical Research Ed.)* 289, no. 6444 (1984): 539–542.

42. Jeannette Pols and Sarah Limburg, "A Matter of Taste? Quality of Life in Day-to-Day Living with ALS and a Feeding Tube," *Culture, Medicine, and Psychiatry* 40, no. 3 (2016): 364.

43. Vincenzo Silani, Edward J. Kasarskis, and Nobuo Yanagisawa, "Nutritional Management in Amyotrophic Lateral Sclerosis: A Worldwide Perspective," *Journal of Neurology* 245, no. 2 (1998): S13–S19.

44. Edward D. Sivak, W. Terry Gipson, and Maurice R. Hanson, "Long-Term Management of Respiratory Failure in Amyotrophic Lateral Sclerosis," *Annals of Neurology* 12, no. 1 (1982): 20.

45. Sivak, Gipson, and Hanson, "Long-Term Management of Respiratory Failure," 20.

46. Sivak, Gipson, and Hanson, "Long-Term Management of Respiratory Failure."

47. Sivak, Gipson, and Hanson, "Long-Term Management of Respiratory Failure," 22.

48. Sivak, Gipson, and Hanson, "Long-Term Management of Respiratory Failure."

49. Hiroshi Mitsumoto and Forbes Holten Norris, *Amyotrophic Lateral Sclerosis: A Comprehensive Guide to Management* (New York: Demos, 1994), 148.

50. Yumiko Kawaguchi, "Impact of the Japanese Disability Homecare System on ALS Patients' Decision to Receive Tracheostomy with Invasive Ventilation," *Neuroethics* 13, no. 2 (2020): 244.

51. Kawaguchi, "Impact of the Japanese Disability Homecare System," 239.

52. Kawaguchi, "Impact of the Japanese Disability Homecare System," 242.

53. Kawaguchi, "Impact of the Japanese Disability Homecare System."

54. M. C. Rousseau, S. Pietra, J. Blaya, and A. Catala, "Quality of Life of ALS and LIS Patients with and without Invasive Mechanical Ventilation," *Journal of Neurology* 258, no. 10 (2011): 1801–1804.

55. David J. Pierson, "History and Epidemiology of Noninvasive Ventilation in the Acute-Care Setting," *Respiratory Care* 54, no. 1 (2009): 40–52.

56. Pierson, "History and Epidemiology of Noninvasive Ventilation."

57. H. L. Motley, L. Werko, A. Cournand, and D. W. Richards, "Observations on the Clinical Use of Intermittent Positive Pressure," *Journal of Aviation Medicine* 18, no. 5 (1947): 417–435.

58. J. Dorst and A. C. Ludolph, "Non-invasive Ventilation in Amyotrophic Lateral Sclerosis," *Therapeutic Advances in Neurological Disorders* 12 (2019): 1–14.

59. David S. Greer and Vincent Mor, "How Medicare Is Altering the Hospice Movement," *Hastings Center Report* 15, no. 5 (1985): 5–9.

60. Abigail Lawlis Kuzma, "Hospice: The Legal Ramifications of a Place to Die," *Indiana Law Journal* 56, no. 4 (1980–1981): 673–702.

61. Greer and Mor, "How Medicare Is Altering the Hospice Movement," 5–6.

62. Greer and Mor, "How Medicare Is Altering the Hospice Movement," 6.

4. ALS CLINIC

1. Nicolas Dodier and Janine Barbot, "La force des dispositifs," *Annales : Histoire, sciences sociales* 71, no. 2 (2016): 422.

2. Dodier and Janine Barbot, "La force des dispositifs," 422.

3. François Flahault, *La parole intermédiaire* (Paris: Seuil, 1978), 38–53. Cf. Oswald Ducrot, *Dire et ne pas dire* (Paris: Hermann, 1972).

4. Theresa Mehl, Berit Jordan, and Stephan Zierz, "'Patients with Amyotrophic Lateral Sclerosis (ALS) Are Usually Nice Persons'—How Physicians Experienced in ALS See the Personality Characteristics of Their Patients," *Brain and Behavior* 7, no. 1 (2017): e00599.

5. PALLIATIVE CARE CLINIC

1. Michel Callon, "An Essay on Framing and Overflowing: Economic Externalities Revisited by Sociology," *Sociological Review* 46, no. 1 (1998): 244–269.

2. Marilyn Strathern, "The Whole Person and Its Artifacts," *Annual Review of Anthropology* 33 (2004): 8.

3. This is an experimental bone marrow–derived mesenchymal stem cell therapy, in which autologous MSCs are induced in culture to produce and deliver neurotrophic factors (NTFs). At the time, it is in phase III trials.

6. EPISTLES TO ONES

1. Frances McGill, *Go Not Gently: Letters from a Patient with Amyotrophic Lateral Sclerosis* (New York: Arno Press 1980), 11.

2. McGill, *Go Not Gently*, 6.

3. McGill, *Go Not Gently*, 6–7.

4. Peter Sloterdijk, "Rules for the Human Zoo: A Response to the Letter on Humanism," *Environment and Planning D: Society and Space* 27, no. 1 (2009): 12–28.

5. Sloterdijk, "Rules for the Human Zoo," 12.

6. Charles Rycroft, "Working Through," in *A Critical Dictionary of Psychoanalysis* (New York: Basic Books, 1968), 179.

7. McGill, *Go Not Gently*, 9.

8. McGill, *Go Not Gently*, 33.

9. McGill, *Go Not Gently*, 33.

10. McGill, *Go Not Gently*, 9.

11. McGill, *Go Not Gently*, 9.

12. McGill, *Go Not Gently*, 12.

13. McGill, *Go Not Gently*, 13.

14. McGill, *Go Not Gently*, 13.

15. McGill, *Go Not Gently*, 13.

16. McGill, *Go Not Gently*, 12.

17. McGill, *Go Not Gently*, 14.

18. This would be a Kleinian and specifically non-Freudian position, to the degree that Freud did not consider it possible for the human being to have a primary anxiety toward death since the subject's unconscious does not accept, in his view, its own mortality. Rachel B. Blass, "On 'the Fear of Death' as the Primary Anxiety: How and Why Klein Differs from Freud," *International Journal of Psychoanalysis* 95, no. 4 (2014): 613–627.

19. McGill, *Go Not Gently*, 7.

20. McGill, *Go Not Gently*, 42.

21. McGill, *Go Not Gently*, 19.

22. McGill, *Go Not Gently*, 32.

23. McGill, *Go Not Gently*, 23.

24. McGill, *Go Not Gently*, 23.

25. McGill, *Go Not Gently*, 24.

26. McGill, *Go Not Gently*, 24.

27. McGill, *Go Not Gently*, 33.

28. McGill, *Go Not Gently*, 31.

29. McGill, *Go Not Gently*, 31.

30. McGill, *Go Not Gently*, 31–33.

31. McGill, *Go Not Gently*, 31–33.

32. McGill, *Go Not Gently*, 31–33.

33. McGill, *Go Not Gently*, 43.

34. McGill, *Go Not Gently*, 43.

35. McGill, *Go Not Gently*, 45.

36. McGill, *Go Not Gently*, 50–53.

37. McGill, *Go Not Gently*, 52.

38. McGill, *Go Not Gently*, 50.

39. McGill, *Go Not Gently*, 51.

40. McGill, *Go Not Gently*, 53.

41. McGill, *Go Not Gently*, 53.

42. Cited (anonymously) in Aubrey Lieberman and D. Frank Benson, "Control of Emotional Expression in Pseudobulbar Palsy: A Personal Experience," *Archives of Neurology* 34, no. 11 (1977): 717–719.

43. McGill, *Go Not Gently*, 56.

44. McGill, *Go Not Gently*, 56.

45. McGill, *Go Not Gently*, 60.

46. McGill, *Go Not Gently*, 75.

47. McGill, *Go Not Gently*, 75.

48. McGill, *Go Not Gently*, 76.

49. McGill, *Go Not Gently*, 76.

50. McGill, *Go Not Gently*, 60.

51. McGill, *Go Not Gently*, 76.

52. McGill, *Go Not Gently*, 77.

53. Lieberman and Benson, "Control of Emotional Expression in Pseudobulbar Palsy."

54. McGill, *Go Not Gently*, 89.

55. The ram's horn, blown at the end of Yom Kippur, the Day of Atonement, the day on which, according to the Jewish tradition, God seals each person's fate for the coming year, in the book of life.

56. McGill, *Go Not Gently*, 89.

57. McGill, *Go Not Gently*, 90.

58. McGill, *Go Not Gently*, 90.

59. McGill, *Go Not Gently*, 90.

60. McGill, *Go Not Gently*, 90.

61. McGill, *Go Not Gently*, 95.

62. McGill, *Go Not Gently*, 96.

63. McGill, *Go Not Gently*, 96.

64. McGill, *Go Not Gently*, 98.

65. McGill, *Go Not Gently*, 99.

66. McGill, *Go Not Gently*, 102.

8. ADVOCATE

1. Brian Wallach, "Congressional Testimony," April 9, 2019, https://iamals.org/i-am-als-co-founder-urges-congress-to-increase-research-funding-for-als/.

2. Regarding the failure in Huntington's research, I am grateful to Dr. Allan Tobin for our discussions on this topic in Paris in 2017 during his research visits at the Centre de Sociologie de l'Innovation.

3. US Department of Health and Human Services, Food and Drug Administration, Center for Drug Evaluation and Research (CDER), Center for Biologics Evaluation and Research (CBER), "Amyotrophic Lateral Sclerosis: Developing Drugs for Treatment Guidance for Industry," September 2019, https://www.fda.gov/regulatory-information /search-fda-guidance-documents/amyotrophic-lateral-sclerosis-developing-drugs -treatment-guidance-industry.

4. https://ir.brainstorm-cell.com/2020-11-17-BrainStorm-Announces-Topline-Results -from-NurOwn-R-Phase-3-ALS-Study.

CONCLUSION

1. Reinhart Koselleck, "'Space of Experience' and 'Horizon of Expectation': Two Historical Categories," in *Futures Past: On the Semantics of Historical Time*, trans. Keith Tribe (New York: Columbia University Press, 2004 [1979]), 261–262.

2. Koselleck, "'Space of Experience' and 'Horizon of Expectation,'" 262–263.

3. Haud Guéguen, and Laurent Jeanpierre, *La perspective du possible: Comment penser ce qui peut nous arriver, et ce que nous pouvons faire* (Paris: La Découverte, 2022), 11.

Index